KETO CHAFFLE

RECIPES COOKBOOK #2020:

500 Quick & Easy, Mouth-watering,

Low-Carb Waffles to Lose Weight with taste and

maintain your Ketogenic Diet

By

Wilda Buckley

TABLE OF CONTENTS

DESCRIPTION

Love to eat waffles but doing a diet now? Look what we got here.

If you have your waffle machine in your kitchen then you need to bring it out and use it while reading this book. If you don't have yet, this is the time to buy it.

A chaffle, or cheddar waffle, is a keto waffle made with eggs and cheddar. Chaffles are turning into an exceptionally well-known keto/low-carb nibble.

You can concoct a chaffle utilizing a waffle iron or smaller than expected waffle producer. The cook time is just a couple of moments, and on the off chance that you cook the chaffle right, you end up with a firm, gooey, flavorful bread/waffle elective.

Chaffles are turning into somewhat of fever with supporters of the keto diet. They're less fastidious about making than most keto bread plans and they're anything but difficult to customize. You can transform the fundamental formula for a chaffle into your creation, extending from appetizing to sweet and anything in the middle. You can likewise change the sort of cheddar you use, creating significant changes in the flavor and surface of the chaffle. Cheddar and mozzarella cheddar are the two most rational decisions, yet you can likewise include parmesan, cream cheddar, or whatever other cheddar that melts well.

You'll get two chaffles out of an enormous egg and about a large portion of a cup of cheddar. Contingent upon the cheddar you use, your calories and net carb tally will change a smidgen. Be that as it may, when all is said in done, accepting you utilize genuine, entire milk cheddar like cheddar or mozzarella (instead of cream cheddar or American cheddar), chaffles are altogether without a carb. Standard serving size of two chaffles contains generally: 300 calories 0g complete carbs 0g net carbs 20g protein 23g fat

As should be obvious, chaffles are about as keto as the formula can be: high-fat, high-protein, and zero-carb. They even work on the meat-eater diet, if you eat cheddar.

While the ketogenic diet is a diet that provides a very low intake of carbohydrates and a high content of proteins and, above all, of fats. A drastic reduction of carbohydrates for the benefit of other nutrients aims to force the body to use fats as a source of energy, with the aim of promoting weight loss. The name "ketogenic" derives from the fact that this diet, by significantly reducing the intake of carbohydrates, leads to the formation of the so-called ketone bodies.

This book cover

- What Is A Chaffle? Why Chaffles? Why Chaffles Well Fit With A Keto Regime?
- How To Make Chaffle
- 11 Tips For Making Delicious and Crispy Chaffles
- Basic Chaffles
- Sandwich Chaffles
- Dessert Chaffles
- Savory Chaffles

And much MORE!

Excited on how to do the different flavor of Chaffles? I know that feeling too! I am on a diet and I love making chaffles every day and night. All of that is because of this book, try it now. Click the buy button and start to make your chaffles too!

INTRODUCTION

General overview of the Keto diet

What is Keto diet?

The word keto is short for ketogenic. The Ketogenic diet focuses on consuming very low amounts of carbohydrates, high levels of fat, and adequate levels of protein. In simple terms, with the Keto diet, you replace carbohydrates with fat. In case you haven't figured this out, carbohydrates are known as carbs, for short. You're probably wondering: The aim of a diet is to lose weight and not to gain more. How does that happen if I'm replacing carbs with fat? It is quite simple, really. When the levels of carbs in your body start to dwindle, your body goes into a metabolic state. This metabolic state is referred to as ketosis. The ketosis state is one in which the body burns fat much more rapidly to convert it into energy. The fat is not only turned to energy but is also turned into ketones. Ketones located in the liver also boost energy. In summary, Keto changes your body's mode of operation. Rather than converting your carbohydrates into energy, the fats you want to rid your body of are converted and burned off instead. The end result of a Keto diet is burned fat, boosted energy, reduced insulin levels, and reduced blood sugar.

Advantages of the Keto diet

The Keto diet has been proven to have many advantages for people over 50. Here are some of the best.

Strengthens bones

When people get older, their bones weaken. At 50, your bones are likely not as strong as they used to be. However, you can keep them in really good condition. Consuming milk to get calcium cannot do enough to strengthen your bones. What you can do, is to make use of the Keto diet as it is low in toxins. Toxins negatively affect the absorption of nutrients and so with this, your bones can take in all they need.

Eradicates inflammation

Few things are worse than the pain from an inflamed joint or muscle. Arthritis, for instance, can be extremely difficult to bear. When you follow the ketosis diet, the production of cytokines will be reduced. Cytokines cause inflammation and therefore, their eradication will reduce it.

It eradicates nutrients deficiency

Keto focuses on consuming exactly what you need. If you use a great Keto plan, your body will lack no nutrients and will not suffer any deficiency.

Reduced hunger

The reason we find it difficult to stick to diets is hunger. It doesn't matter your age; diets do not become easier. We may have a mental picture of the healthy body we want. We may even have clear visuals of the kind of life we want to lead once free from unhealthy living but none of that matters when hunger enters the scene. However, the Keto diet is a diet that combats this problem. The Keto diet focuses on consuming plenty of proteins. Proteins are filling and do not let you feel hungry too easily. In addition, when your carb levels are reduced, your appetite takes a hit. It is a win-win situation.

Weight loss

Keto not only burns fat, but it also reduces that craving for food. Combined, these are two great ways to lose weight. It is one of the diets that has proven to help the most when it comes to weight loss. The Keto diet has been proven to be one of the best ways to burn stubborn belly fat while keeping yourself revitalized and healthy.

Reduces blood sugar and insulin

After 50, monitoring blood sugar can be a real struggle. Cutting down on carbs drastically reduces both insulin levels and blood sugar levels. This means that the Keto diet will benefit millions as a lot of people struggle with insulin complications and high blood sugar levels. It has been proven to help as when some people embark on Keto, they cut up to half of the carbs they consume. It's a treasure for those with diabetes and insulin resistance. A study was carried out on people with type 2 diabetes. After cutting down on carbs, within six months, 95 percent of people were able to reduce or totally stop using their glucose-lowering medication.

Lower levels of triglycerides

A lot of people do not know what triglycerides are. Triglycerides are molecules of fat in your blood. They are known to circulate the bloodstream and can be very dangerous. High levels of triglycerides can cause heart failures and heart diseases. However, Keto is known to reduce these levels.

Reduces acne

Although acne is mostly suffered by those who are young, there are cases of people above 50 having it. Moreover, Keto is not only for persons after 50. Acne is not only caused by blocked pores. There are quite a number of things proven to cause it. One of these things is your blood sugar. When you consume processed and refined carbs, it affects gut bacteria and results in the fluctuation of blood sugar levels. When the gut bacteria and sugar levels are affected, the skin suffers. However, when you embark on the Keto diet, you cut off on carbs intake which means that in the very first place, your gut bacteria will not be affected thereby cutting off that avenue to develop.

Increases hdl levels

HDL refers to high-density lipoprotein. When your HDL levels are compared to your LDL levels and are not found low, your risk of developing a heart disease is lowered. This is great for persons over 50 as heart diseases suddenly become more probable. Eating fats and reducing your intake of carbohydrates is one of the most assured ways to increase your high-density lipoprotein levels.

Reduces ldl levels

High levels of LDL can be very problematic when you attain 50. This is because LDL refers to bad cholesterol. People with high levels of this cholesterol are more likely to get heart attacks. When you reduce the number of carbs you consume, you will increase the size of bad LDL particles. However, this will result in the reduction of the total LDL particles as they would have increased in size. Smaller LDL particles have been linked to heart diseases while larger ones have been proven to have lower risks attached.

May help combat cancer

I termed this under 'may' because research on this is not as extensive and conclusive as we would like it to be. However, there is proof supporting it. Firstly, it helps reduce the levels of blood sugar which in turn reduces insulin complications which in turn reduces the risk of developing cancers related to insulin levels. In addition, Keto places more oxidative stress on cancer cells than on normal cells thereby making it great for chemotherapy. The risk of developing cancer after fifty is still existent and so, Keto is literally a lifesaver.

May lower blood pressure

High blood pressure plagues adults much more than it does young ones. Once you attain 50, you must monitor your blood pressure rates. Reduction in the intake of carbohydrates is a proven way to lower your blood pressure. When you cut down on your carbs and lower your blood sugar levels, you greatly reduce your chances of getting some other diseases.

Combats metabolic syndrome

As you grow older, you may find that you struggle to control your blood sugar level. Metabolic syndrome is another condition that has been proven to have an influence on diabetes and heart disease development. The symptoms associated with metabolic syndrome include but are not limited to high triglycerides, obesity, high blood sugar level, and low levels of high-density lipoprotein cholesterol.

However, you will find that reducing your level of carbohydrate intake greatly affects this. You will improve your health and majorly attack all the above-listed symptoms. Keto diet helps to fight against metabolic syndrome which is a big win.

Great for the heart

People over the age of 50 have been proven to have more chances of developing heart diseases. Keto diet has been proven to be great for the heart. As it increases good cholesterol levels and reduces the levels of bad cholesterol, you will find that partaking in the Keto diet proves extremely beneficial for your health.

May reduce seizure risks

When you change your intake levels the combination of protein, fat, and carbs, as we explained before, your body will go into ketosis. Ketosis has been proven to reduce seizure levels in people who suffer from epilepsy. When they do not respond to treatment, the ketosis treatment is used. This has been done for decades.

Combats brain disorders

Keto doesn't end there, it also combats Alzheimer's and Parkinson's disease. There are some parts of your brain that can only burn glucose and so, your body needs it. If you do not consume carbs, your lover will make use of protein to produce glucose. Your brain can also burn ketones. Ketones are formed when your carb level is very low. With this, the ketogenic diet has been used f r plenty of years to treat epilepsy in children who aren't responding to drugs. For adults, it can work the same magic as it is now being linked to treating Alzheimer's and Parkinson's disease

Helps women suffering from polycystic ovarian syndrome (pcos)

This syndrome affects women of all ages. PCOS is short for polycystic ovarian syndrome. Polycystic ovarian syndrome is an endocrine disorder that results in enlarged ovaries with cysts.

These cysts are dangerous and cause other complications. It has been proven that a high intake of carbohydrates negatively affects women suffering from polycystic ovarian syndrome. When a woman with PCOS cuts down on carbs and embarks on the Keto diet, the polycystic ovarian syndrome falls under attack.

It is beyond doubt that the Keto diet is beneficial in so many ways that it almost looks unreal. If you are to embark on the Keto diet, there are several things you must know.

Caution for Keto

Yes, Keto is beneficial and yes, it has a lot of benefits but it is no small thing and so, it must be approached with caution. Here are some tips you should keep in mind before embarking on Keto.

Make use of recipes you can trust

Keto involves a lot of meal planning and this single phase is where a lot of people get it wrong. Your meals are no longer allowed to be careless and you must note everything that goes into your mouth. If you are embarking on a Keto diet, you must use recipes you can trust. The recipes must be beneficial, safe, and delicious. Keto should not take out the enjoyment in your meals. Luckily, you have your hands on the best book for Keto aspirants under 50.

You may need a doctor

If you have had any issue with blood sugar, insulin levels or diabetes, consult your doctor before embarking on Keto. Do not make any dietary changes as large as Keto to your diet without first informing your doctor. He or she is in the best position to guide you properly. See your doctor.

It will be hard at first

Keto is no walk in the park. However, people continue on the path of Keto despite the initial difficulty because the results are evident after a short while. When you kick-start Keto, you may suffer from low blood sugar, sluggishness, and constipation, However, they will all wear off in a few days if you are religious about it.

Can Keto have side effects?

Yes. Keto can have side effects. Keto can have negative side effects if it is wrongly done. Keto cuts down on carbs and replaces them with fat. However, if the replacement is not adequately carried out, a lot of negative side effects may occur. This is why it is extremely important to begin the Keto diet armed with the right information and recipes which are all included in this book.

If you do not make use of quality meal plans and recipes, you'll lack nutrients that your body needs. With Keto, you must not lack proteins and so, your meals must be planned.

How to reach ketosis

Reaching the state of ketosis is not so straightforward for many people. In order to effectively reach ketosis, there are some steps you must take.

Eat the right food- Ketosis relies a lot on what you eat. To reach ketosis, you need to first cut down on the carbohydrates you take in. Secondly, you need to take in much more fats in your diets. However, you should just take in any fat, you should make sure to take in healthy fat. Taking in unhealthy fats can cause more harm than good.

Exercise- To efficiently reach ketosis, you should make sure to exercise. It doesn't have to be intensive, however, long walks, jugs, biking, and other exercises can help your body reach ketosis.

Try intermittent fasting- Some people combine intermittent fasting with ketosis. The reason is that, as you progress, your hunger pangs are reduced greatly and you will find intermittent fasting easy. In fact, even when you do not plan to, you'll find yourself doing it. It is definitely not compulsory but if you are making use of ketosis to lose weight, intermittent fasting is a great bonus.

Take lots of fruits and vegetables- Fruits and vegetables for snacks will keep your body healthy and help revitalize your skin.

Include coconut oil in your diet- Coconut is compulsory if you want to reach ketosis. Coconut oil contains healthy fat. It helps the body reach ketosis and contains four types of MCTs. It is one of the best tools for inducing ketosis. If you have never made use of coconut oil before, start slowly and increase your intake gradually.

WHAT IS A CHAFFLE? WHY CHAFFLES? WHY CHAFFLES WELL FIT WITH A KETO REGIME?

The Meaning Of Chaffle

Chaffles (short for cheddar waffles) are the most recent famous nourishment in the keto world. It's nothing unexpected — the chaffle has a great deal putting it all on the line. This straightforward keto formula is fresh, brilliant dark colored, sans sugar, low-carb, and exceptionally simple to make.

A chaffle, or cheddar waffle, is a keto waffle made with eggs and cheddar. Chaffles are turning into an extremely well known keto/low-carb nibble.

A chaffle is a waffle yet made with a cheddar base. Basically it's obliterated cheddar and an egg mix. Once in for a short time for logically fluffier recipes, it's a cream cheddar base instead of decimated cheddar. It's the a la mode new keto-pleasing bread since it's low in carbs, and it won't spike your insulin levels, causing fat accumulating.

The fundamentals are some combo of egg and cheddar; however, from here, you can riff like wild eyed. You can use an arrangement of cheeses, including cream cheddar, parmesan cheddar, etc. Some incorporate almond flour and flaxseed and getting ready powder, and others don't.

The major recipe for a chaffle contains cheddar, almond flour, and an egg. You consolidate the fixings in an astonish and pour it your waffle maker. Waffle makers are no doubt on the rising right now after this chaffle recipe exploded a couple of days back earlier. I was to some degree suspicious from the beginning intuition there was no possibility this would turn out in the wake of joining everything and pouring the hitter over the waffle. Try to sprinkle the waffle maker really well. The waffle wound up exceptional, and it was firm apparently and fragile in the inside.

You can concoct a chaffle utilizing a waffle iron or smaller than usual waffle producer. The cook time is just a couple of moments, and on the off chance that you cook the chaffle right, you end up with a fresh, gooey, flavorful bread/waffle elective.

Chaffles are turning into somewhat of a furor with supporters of the keto diet. They're less fastidious to make than most keto bread recipes and they're anything but difficult to customize. You can transform the fundamental formula for a chaffle into your own creation, running from flavorful to sweet and anything in the middle. You can likewise change the sort of cheddar you use, delivering significant changes in the flavor and surface of the chaffle. Cheddar and mozzarella cheddar are the two most regular decisions, yet you can likewise include parmesan, cream cheddar, or whatever other cheddar that melts well.

The most fundamental clarification of a Chaffle is that it's an extraordinary bread elective when on the keto diet. It copies the vibe of a waffle however Keto clients have been utilizing Chaffles in a wide range of recipes from sandwiches to sweets. There are a huge amount of Keto Chaffle Recipes out there.

It's made with cheddar, so get it? At the point when you work cheddar and waffle – you get chaffle (and you additionally get enchantment.) Well enough with the back story. Since you realize what this keto nourishment is, how about we make one and let you see with your own eyes how astounding this keto waffle is.

Chaffles Nutrition and Carb Count

You'll get two chaffles out of an enormous egg and about a large portion of a cup of cheddar. Contingent upon the cheddar you use, your calories and net carb check will change a tad. Yet, as a rule, expecting you utilize genuine, entire milk cheddar like cheddar or mozzarella (rather than cream cheddar or American cheddar), chaffles are totally sans carb. A normal serving size of two chaffles contains generally:

300 calories

0g all out carbs

0g net carbs

20g protein

23g fat

As should be obvious, chaffles are about as keto as a formula can be: high-fat, high-protein, and zero-carb. They even work on the flesh eater diet, if you eat cheddar.

HOW TO MAKE CHAFFLE

What Is Needed To Prepare A Chaffle

1 tremendous egg

1/2 c. Cheddar

2 tablespoons of almond flour

How To Prepare A Chaffle

There are a few hints, techniques and approaches you'll need to know to make your chaffles particularly fresh.

Most importantly, don't eat your chaffles directly out of the waffle iron. They'll be wet and eggy from the outset, however on the off chance that you let them sit for 3-4 minutes, they'll fresh right up.

Second, for extra fresh chaffles, you can include an additional layer of destroyed cheddar (or another cheddar that gets firm, similar to parmesan) to the two sides of the waffle producer's surface. Set out the destroyed cheddar, pour in the hitter, put more cheddar on top, and afterward cook the chaffle typically. You'll wind up with firm, sautéed bits of cheddar installed in the outside of the chaffle.

Everyone is going looney tunes, asking, "How might I make these?!" This is the game plan The principal recipe on what and how. The fundamental equation consolidates crushed cheddar and an egg; however, there are tremendous measures of add-ins you can use to change the flavor! You will make a direct chaffle hitter and cook it in a waffle maker!

To make a chaffle equation, you will fundamentally join two or three fixings and cook it in a waffle maker to make a perfect work of art everyone will value!

1. Preheat your waffle maker if it requires preheating.

2. Whisk together the egg, cheddar, almond flour, and setting up the soda pop in a bowl until all-around joined.

3. Shower the waffle maker with a cooking sprinkle and pour the chaffle player over the waffle maker. Close and let the waffle for 3 to 4 minutes. My waffle maker has it's own customized clock setting.

4. Remove the waffle from the waffle press and welcome it.

5. The Waffle Tools To Make Easy Keto Chaffles

A standard waffle creator will deliver a chaffle that appears as though the universally adored round solidified toaster waffles, which is flawless as keto bread for sandwiches, a bun for burgers, or even a shell for tacos. One famous brand is the Dash smaller than expected waffle creator, which is entirely reasonable and makes slender, fresh chaffles.

A Belgian waffle creator makes thicker waffles with profound scores. That is incredible for typical waffle-production, however it isn't perfect for chaffles. They end up less fresh, with a greater amount of an omelet-like consistency. Your most logical option is to get a standard waffle producer.

How To Eat Chaffles

There are a great deal of famous approaches to eat chaffles.

- Plain. Chaffles are incredible all alone as a morning meal nourishment. You can serve them up close by bacon, eggs, avocado, and other standard keto breakfast passage.

- Keto chaffle sandwich. Make two chaffles and use them as bread for your preferred sandwich. Chaffles are extraordinary as the bread for BLTs, turkey clubs, breakfast sandwiches, or some other keto-accommodating sandwich.

- Chaffle dessert. Attempt one of the sweet chaffle varieties recorded underneath and present with keto maple syrup or your most loved keto frozen yogurt.

The Various Types Of Basic Keto Chaffle Recipes

Keto Chaffle Recipes eBook Cookbook for beginners 2020, includes delicious and appealing keto recipes for each flavor palette.

1. Basic Chaffle Recipes
2. Savory Chaffle Recipes
3. Sweet Chaffle Recipes
4. Chaffle Cake Recipes

Various Cheeses

Cheddar, mozzarella, parmesan, cream cheddar, colby jack — any cheddar that melts well will work with a chaffle. Distinctive cheddar produce various flavors and somewhat various surfaces. Attempt a couple and locate your top choice.

Sweet Chaffles

Utilize a nonpartisan cheddar like mozzarella or cream cheddar, at that point include a touch of your most loved keto sugar to the hitter before you cook it. You can likewise chocolate chips or low-sugar fruits like blueberries or strawberries. Top with keto frozen yogurt or keto whipped cream for a delectable chaffle dessert.

Exquisite Chaffles

Include exquisite fixings like herbs and flavors to your chaffle. For a pizza chaffle, include oregano, garlic powder, and diced pepperoni in the hitter, with tomato sauce and additional cheddar on top. Or on the other hand you could utilize cream cheddar and add everything bagel flavoring to the player for an everything bagel chaffle. Present with more cream cheddar on top, tricks, onions, and smoked salmon.

11 TIPS FOR MAKING
DELICIOUS AND CRISPY CHAFFLES

1. Start making chaffles with the basic mini waffle maker.

2. Don't overfill the mini waffle maker, use 1/8-1/4 cup of batter

3. Spray waffle maker with coconut oil before cooking for a crispy texture.

4. A layer of cheese before and after the batter in maker can give it a crispy texture. Sprinkling 1 tbsp. cheese before and after the batter in the waffle maker may help to release chaffles easily from waffle maker and makes chaffles crunchy.

5. Always preheat waffle maker before cookingso that it will be less sticky and easier to clean up.

6. Instead of using the whole egg, egg whites can be used in chaffles to give it no eggy flavor.

7. Let chaffles stand at room temperature to give it a crunchy texture.

8. Do not fill waffle maker with more than 1/4 cup of TOTAL ingredients at a time.

9. Use a wet paper towel to clean up the waffle maker when the waffle iron is warm to clean it easily.

10. Use a toothbrush to clean inside the waffle machine.

11. Use shredded cheese instead of a slice in the batter. It helps to mix all ingredients well.

BASIC CHAFFLES

1. Fluffy Keto Chaffle

Preparation Time: 3 min
Cooking Time: 4 min
Servings: 1

Ingredients

- egg
- 1/2 cup cheddar cheese, shredded

Directions:

1- Switch on the waffle maker according to manufacturer's instructions

2- Crack egg and combine with cheddar cheese in a small bowl

3- Place half batter on waffle maker and spread evenly.

4- Cook for 4 minutes or until as desired

5- Gently remove from waffle maker and set aside for 2 minutes so it cools down and become crispy

6- Repeat for remaining batter

7- Serve with desired toppings

2. Keto Sandwich Chaffle

Preparation Time: 3 min
Cooking Time: 4 min
Servings: 1

Ingredients

- 1 egg
- 1/2 cup cheddar cheese, shredded
- 1 tbsp almond flour (optional)

Directions:

1. Using a mini waffle maker, preheat according to maker's instructions.

2. Combine egg and cheddar cheese in a mixing bowl. Stir thoroughly

3. Add Almond flour for added texture if so desired

4. Place half batter on waffle maker and spread evenly.

5. Cook for 4 minutes or until as desired

6. Gently remove from waffle maker and set aside for 2 minutes so it cools down and become crispy

7. Repeat for remaining batter

8. Stuff 2 chaffles with garnishing to make a sandwich

03. Traditional Chaffle

Preparation Time: 5 min
Cooking Time: 4 min
Servings: 2 mini waffles

Ingredients:

- 1 large egg
- 1/2 cup finely shredded mozzarella

Directions:

1. Switch on the mini waffle maker according to manufacturer's instructions

2. Spray the waffle iron with non-stick spray

3. Crack egg and combine with cheddar cheese in a small bowl

4. Place half batter on waffle maker and spread evenly.

5. Cook for 4 minutes or until as desired

6. Gently remove from waffle maker and set aside for 2 minutes so it cools down and become crispy

7. Repeat with remaining batter.

8. Serve warm with desired toppings (optional) - butter, strawberries and sugar-free syrup

04.Fluffy Sandwich Breakfast Chaffle

Preparation Time: 5 min
Cooking Time: 3 min
Servings: 2

Ingredients:

- 1/2 tsp Psyllium husk powder (optional)
- tbsp almond flour
- 1/4 tsp Baking powder (optional)
- 1 large Egg
- 1/2 cup Mozzarella cheese, shredded
- 1 tbsp vanilla or
- Dash of cinnamon

Directions:

1. Switch on the waffle maker according to manufacturer's instructions
2. Crack egg and combine with cheddar cheese in a small bowl
3. Add remaining ingredients and combine thoroughly.
4. Place half batter on waffle maker and spread evenly.
5. Cook for 4 minutes or until as desired
6. Gently remove from waffle maker and set aside for 2 minutes so it cools down and become crispy
7. Repeat for remaining batter
8. Serve with keto ice cream topping

05.Keto Plain Prepped Chaffles

Preparation Time: 3 min
Cooking Time: 6 min
Servings: 1

Ingredients

- small eggs
- 1/2 cup shredded cheddar cheese

Directions:

1. Preheat mini waffle maker until hot
2. Whisk egg in a bowl, add cheese, then mix well
3. Stir in the remaining ingredients (except toppings, if any).
4. Grease waffle maker and Scoop 1/2 of the batter onto the waffle maker, spread across evenly
5. Cook until a bit browned and crispy, about 4 minutes.
6. Gently remove from waffle maker and let it cool
7. Repeat with remaining batter.
8. Store in the fridge for 3-5 days.

06.Vanilla Keto Chaffle

Preparation Time: 3 min
Cooking Time: 4 min
Servings: 1

Ingredients

- 1 egg
- 1/2 cup cheddar cheese, shredded
- 1/2 tsp vanilla extract

Directions

1. Switch on the waffle maker according to manufacturer's instructions
2. Crack egg and combine with cheddar cheese in a small bowl
3. Add vanilla extract and combine thoroughly.
4. Place half batter on waffle maker and spread evenly.
5. Cook for 4 minutes or until as desired

6. Gently remove from waffle maker and set aside for 2 minutes so it cools down and become crispy

7. Repeat for remaining batter

07.Crispy Sandwich Chaffle

Preparation Time: 3 min
Cooking Time: 4 min
Servings: 1

Ingredients

- 1 egg
- 1/2 cup cheddar cheese, shredded
- 1 tbsp coconut flour

Directions:

1. Using a mini waffle maker, preheat according to maker's instructions.

2. Combine egg and cheddar cheese in a mixing bowl. Stir thoroughly

3. Add coconut flour for added texture if so desired

4. Place half batter on waffle maker and spread evenly.

5. Cook for 4 minutes or until as desired

6. Gently remove from waffle maker and set aside for 2 minutes so it cools down and become crispy

7. Repeat for remaining batter

8. Stuff 2 chaffles with desired sandwich

08.Basic Keto Chaffle

Preparation Time: 3 min
Cooking Time: 4 min
Servings: 1

Ingredients

- 1 egg
- 1/2 cup cheddar cheese, shredded
- 1/2 tbsp Psyllium husk powder

- 1/2 tbsp chia seeds

Directions:

1. Switch on the waffle maker according to manufacturer's instructions

2. Crack egg and combine with cheddar cheese in a small bowl

3. Place half batter on waffle maker and spread evenly.

4. Sprinkle Chia on top, cover and cook for 4 minutes or until as desired

5. Gently remove from waffle maker and set aside for 2 minutes so it cools down and become crispy

6. Repeat for remaining batter

7. Serve with desired toppings

09.Keto Sandwich Chaffle

Preparation Time: 3 min
Cooking Time: 4 min
Servings: 1

Ingredients

- 1 egg
- 1/2 cup cheddar cheese, shredded
- 1 tbsp almond flour (optional)

Directions:

1. Using a mini waffle maker, preheat according to maker's instructions.

2. Combine egg and cheddar cheese in a mixing bowl. Stir thoroughly

3. Add Almond flour for added texture if so desired; mix well

4. Place half batter on waffle maker and spread evenly.

5. Cook for 4 minutes or until as desired

6. Gently remove from waffle maker and set aside for 2 minutes so it cools down and become crispy

7. Repeat for remaining batter

8. Stuff 2 chaffles with desired garnishing to make a sandwich

Nutrition:

170 calories
2g net carbs
14g fat
10g protein

10.Flaky Delight Chaffle

Preparation Time: 3 min
Cooking Time: 4 min
Servings: 1

Ingredients

- 1 egg
- 1/2 cup cheddar cheese, shredded
- 1/2 cup coconut flakes

Directions:

1. Switch on the waffle maker according to manufacturer's instructions

2. Crack egg and combine with cheddar cheese in a small bowl

3. Place half batter on waffle maker and spread evenly.

4. Sprinkle coconut flakes and Cook for 4 minutes or until as desired

5. Gently remove from waffle maker and set aside for 2 minutes so it cools down and become crispy

6. Repeat for remaining batter

7. Serve with desired toppings

Nutrition:

291 calories
1g net carbs
23g fat
20g protein

11.Keto Minty Base Chaffle

Preparation Time: 3 min
Cooking Time: 4 min
Servings: 1

Ingredients

- 1 egg
- 1/2 cup cheddar cheese, shredded
- 1 tbsp mint extract (low carb)

Directions:

1. Using a mini waffle maker, preheat according to maker's instructions.

2. Combine egg and cheddar cheese in a mixing bowl. Stir thoroughly

3. Add mint extract and place half batter on waffle maker; spread evenly.

4. Cook for 4 minutes or until as desired

5. Gently remove from waffle maker and set aside for 2 minutes so it cools down and become crispy

6. Repeat for remaining batter

7. Garnish with desired toppings

Nutrition:

170 calories
2g net carbs
14g fat
10g protein

12.Okonomiyaki Chaffle

Preparation time: 22 minutes
Cooking time: 11 minutes
Servings: 2

Ingredients:

- Okonomiyaki Chaffle
- Mozzarella Cheese: ½ cup
- Baking powder: ½ teaspoon
- Egg: 2
- Cabbage: ¼ cup (shredded)

- Sauce
- Soy Sauce: 4 teaspoons
- Swerve/Monk fruit: 2 tablespoons
- Ketchup: 4 tablespoons (sugar-free)
- Worcestershire Sauce: 4 teaspoons
- Toppings
- Kewpie Mayo: 2 tablespoons
- Beni Shoga: 2 tablespoons
- Green Onion: 1 stalk
- Bonito Flakes: 4 tablespoons
- Dried Seaweed Powder: 2 tablespoons

Directions:

1. Prepare a mix of chopped onions and finely cut cabbage and set aside. Using a mixing bowl, prepare another mix for the sauce containing all ingredients for the sauce and also set aside. Quickly, preheat a mini-sized waffle and grease it. In another mixing bowl, prepare a mix of shredded mozzarella cheese with cabbage, beaten eggs and baking powder. Combine the mixture and pour into the lower side of the waffle maker. With the lid closed, cook for 5 minutes to a crunch. Once timed out, take out waffles and serve in a plate. Repeat process for the remaining waffle mixture. Garnish the chaffles with beni shoga, bonito flakes, chopped onions and dried seaweed powder. Pour the prepared sauce with Kewpie mayo. Serve and enjoy.

13.Jalapeno Cheddar Chaffle

Preparation time: 12 minutes
Required cooking time: 5 minutes
Servings: 2

Ingredients:

- Egg: 2

- Deli Jalapeno: 16 slices
- Cheddar cheese: 1½ cup

Directions:

2. Preheat and grease a waffle maker. Prepare a mixture containing ½ half cheddar with beaten eggs, then mix evenly. Sprinkle some shredded cheese at the base of the waffle maker, then pour the batter on the cheese and top again with more cheese with4 slices of Jalapeno. With the lid closed, cook for 5 minutes to a crunch. Repeat the process for the remaining mixture. Serve and enjoy.

14.Bacon Cheddar Chaffle

Preparation time: 12 minutes
Required cooking time: 6 minutes
Servings: 2

Ingredients:

- Egg: 1
- Bacon bite: As per your taste
- Cheddar cheese: 1½ cup

Directions:

1. First, preheat and grease the waffle maker. Prepare a mix of all ingredients in a bowl, then pour into a waffle maker and heat for 4 minutes in a waffle maker until it turns crispy. Repeat the process for the remaining mixture. Serve the dish to enjoy.

15.Simple And Crispy Chaffle

Preparation time: 12 minutes
Required cooking time: 6 minutes
Servings available: 2

Ingredients:

- Cheddar cheese: 1/3 cup
- Baking powder: 1/4 teaspoon

- Parmesan cheese (shredded): 1/3 cup
- Egg: 1
- Flaxseed: 1 teaspoon (ground)

Directions:

1. Prepare a mix containing egg, baking powder, flaxseed, and cheddar seed in a mixing bowl. Preheat and grease the waffle maker. Sprinkle the shredded cheddar cheese at the base of the waffle maker and pour the mixture into the waffle maker, then add some more shredded cheese at the top of the mixture. Heat the mixture to cook to a crispy form. Repeat the process for the remaining mixture. Serve the dish to enjoy.

16.Crispy Zucchini Chaffles

Preparation time: 18 minutes
Required cooking time: 12 minutes
Servings available: 2

Ingredients:

- Zucchini: 1 (small – finely grated)
- Egg: 1
- Shredded mozzarella: half cup
- Parmesan: 1 tablespoon
- Pepper: As per your taste
- Basil: 1 teaspoon

Directions:

1. 1.Preheat and grease the waffle maker. Prepare a mix of all the ingredients in a mixing bowl. Pour the mixture into a large-sized waffle maker and spread evenly. Heat the mixtures to a crunchy form. Repeat the process for the remaining mixture. Serve hot and enjoy the crispy taste.

17.Rich And Creamy Mini Chaffle

Preparation time: 12 minutes
Required cooking time: 6 minutes
Servings available: 2

Ingredients:

- Baking powder: ¾ tablespoon
- Eggs: 2
- Cream cheese: 2 tablespoons
- Almond flour: 2 tablespoons
- Water: 2 tablespoon (optional)
- Shredded mozzarella: 1 cup

Directions:

1. Preheat and grease the waffle maker. Prepare a mix of all the ingredients in a mixing bowl. Pour the mixture into a large-sized waffle maker and spread evenly. Heat the mixtures to a crunchy form for 5 minutes. Repeat the process for the remaining mixture. Serve hot and enjoy the crispy taste.

18.Jalapeno Bacon Swiss Chaffle

Preparation time: 18 minutes
Required cooking time: 12 minutes
Servings available: 2

Ingredients:

- Shredded Swiss cheese: ½ cup
- Fresh jalapenos (diced): 1 tablespoon
- Bacon piece: 2 tablespoon
- Egg: 1

Directions:

1. First, preheat and grease the waffle maker. Using a pan, cook the bacon pieces, put off the heat and shred the cheese and egg. Add in the diced fresh jalapenos and mix evenly. Heat the waffle makers to get the mixture into a crispy form. Repeat the process for

the remaining mixture. Serve the dish to enjoy.

19.Chaffle Tacos

This recipe for Taco Chaffle Shells is easy to make, super crispy, and mouthwateringly delicious.
Preparation time: 5 mins
Cooking time: 8 Mins

Ingredients

- 1 egg white
- 1/4 cup Monterey jack cheese, shredded (packed tightly)
- 1/4 cup sharp cheddar cheese, shredded (packed tightly)
- 3/4 tsp water
- 1 tsp coconut flour
- 1/4 tsp baking powder
- 1/8 tsp chili powder
- Pinch of salt

Directions

1. Plug the Dash Mini Waffle Maker in the wall and grease lightly once it is hot.

2. Combine all of the ingredients in a bowl and stir to combine.

3. Spoon out 1/2 of the batter on the waffle maker and close lid. Set a timer for 4 minutes and do not lift the lid until the cooking time is complete. If you do, it will look like the taco chaffle shell isn't set up properly, but it will. You have to let it cook the entire 4 minutes before lifting the lid.

4. Remove the taco chaffle shell from the waffle iron and set aside. Repeat the same steps above with the rest of the chaffle batter.

5. Turn over a muffin pan and set the taco chaffle shells between the cups to form a taco shell. Allow the setting for a few minutes.

6. Enjoy this delicious keto crispy taco chaffle shell with your favorite toppings.

7. Notes

8. The nutritional information provided is only for the keto taco chaffle shells recipe.

Nutrition

Serving: 2g | Calories: 258kcal | Carbohydrates: 4g | Protein: 18g | Fat: 19g | Fiber: 2g | Sugar: 1g

20.Cheddar Biscuit Chaffle

All the flavor of a Cheddar Bay Biscuit from your favorite lobster restaurant in a keto-approved waffle. The Cheddar Bay Biscuit Chaffle is a delicious mix of savory garlic and cheddar cheese.
Preparation time: 15 minutes
Cooking time: 5 minutes

Ingredients:

- 1 egg
- ¼ cup sharp cheddar cheese
- 2 tablespoons almond flour
- ½ teaspoon baking powder
- ½ teaspoon garlic powder
- pinch of salt

Directions:

1. Preheat waffle maker to medium-high heat.

2. Whisk together egg, cheddar cheese, almond flour, baking powder, garlic powder, and salt.

3. Pour chaffle mixture into the center of the waffle iron. Close the waffle maker and let cook for 3-5 minutes or until waffle is golden brown and set.

4. Remove chaffle from the waffle maker and serve.

21.Keto Blueberry Chaffle

Preparation Time: 3 minutes
Cooking Time: 15 minutes
Servings: 5

Ingredients:

- 1 cup of mozzarella cheese
- 2 tablespoons almond flour
- 1 tsp baking powder
- 2 eggs
- 1 tsp cinnamon
- 2 tsp of Swerve
- tablespoon blueberries

Directions:

1. Heat up your Dash mini waffle maker.

2. In a mixing bowl, add the mozzarella cheese, almond flour, baking powder, eggs, cinnamon, swerve, and blueberries. Mix well, so all the ingredients are mixed together.

3. Spray your mini waffle maker with nonstick cooking spray.

4. Add in a little bit less than 1/4 a cup of blueberry keto waffle batter.

5. Close the lid and cook the chaffle for 3-5 minutes. Check it at the 3-minute mark to see if it is crispy and brown. If it is not or it sticks to the top of the waffle machine, close the lid and cook for 1-2 minutes longer.

6. Serve with a sprinkle of swerve confectioners sugar or keto syrup.

22.Keto Chaffle Taco Shells

Preparation Time: 5 minutes
Cooking Time: 20 minutes
Servings: 5

Ingredients:

- 1 tablespoon almond flour
- 1 cup taco blend cheese
- 2 eggs
- 1/4 tsp taco seasoning

Directions:

1. In a bowl, mix almond flour, taco blend cheese, eggs, and taco seasoning. I find it easiest to mix everything using a fork.

2. Add 1.5 tablespoons of taco chaffle batter to the waffle maker at a time — Cook chaffle batter in the waffle maker for 4 minutes.

3. Remove the taco chaffle shell from the waffle maker and drape over the side of a bowl. I used my pie pan because it was what I had on hand, but just about any bowl will work.

4. Continue making chaffle taco shells until you are out of batter. Then fill your taco shells with taco meat, your favorite toppings, and enjoy!

23.Pumpkin Chocolate Chip Chaffles

Preparation Time: 4 minutes
Cooking Time: 12 minutes
Servings: 3

Ingredients:

- 1/2 cup shredded mozzarella cheese
- teaspoons pumpkin puree
- 1 egg
- 2 tablespoons granulated Swerve
- 1/4 tsp pumpkin pie spice
- 4 teaspoons sugar-free chocolate chips
- 1 tablespoon almond flour

Directions:

1. Plug in your waffle maker.

2. In a small bowl, mix the pumpkin puree and egg. Make sure you mix it well, so all the pumpkin is mixed with the egg.

3. Next, add in the mozzarella cheese, almond flour, swerve and add pumpkin spice and mix well.

4. Then add in your sugar-free chocolate chips

5. Add half the keto pumpkin pie Chaffle mix to the Dish Mini waffle maker at a time. Cook chaffle batter in the waffle maker for 4 minutes.

6. Do not open before the 4 minutes is up. It is very important that you do not open the waffle maker before the 4-minute mark. After that you can open it to check it and make sure it is cooked all the way, but with these chaffles keeping the lid closed the whole time is very important.

7. When the first one is completely done cooking cook the second one.

8. Enjoy with some swerve confectioners sweetener or whipped cream on top.

24.Peanut Butter Chocolate Chip Chaffle

Preparation Time: 2 minutes
Cooking Time: 8 minutes
Servings: 2

Ingredients:

- 1 egg.
- 1/4 cup shredded mozzarella cheese
- 2 tablespoons creamy Peanut Butter.
- 1 tablespoon Almond Flour.
- 1 tablespoon Granulated Swerve.
- 1 teaspoon Vanilla extract.

- 1 tablespoon low carb chocolate chips.

Directions:

1. Plug in your waffle maker.

2. In a small bowl, mix the peanut butter and egg. Make sure you mix it well, so all the peanut butter is mixed with the egg.

3. Next, add in the mozzarella cheese, almond flour, swerve and chocolate chips and mix well.

4. Add half the keto peanut butter chocolate chip Chaffle mix to the Dish Mini waffle maker at a time. Cook chaffle batter in the waffle maker for 4 minutes.

5. When the first one is completely done cooking cook the second one.

6. Enjoy with some swerve confectioners sweetener or whipped cream on top.

25.Broccoli & Cheese Chaffle

Preparation Time: 2 minutes
Cooking Time: 8 minutes
Servings: 2

Ingredients:

- 1/2 cup cheddar cheese
- 1/4 cup fresh chopped broccoli
- 1 egg
- 1/4 teaspoon garlic powder
- 1 tablespoon almond flour

Directions:

1. In a bowl, mix almond flour, cheddar cheese, egg, and garlic powder. I find it easiest to mix everything using a fork.

2. Add half the Broccoli and Cheese Chaffle batter to the Dish Mini waffle maker at a time.

3. Cook chaffle batter in the waffle maker for 4 minutes.

4. Let each chaffle sit for 1-2 minutes on a plate to firm up. Enjoy alone or dipping in sour cream or ranch dressing.

26.Savory Cauliflower Chaffles with Cream Cheese Frosting

Preparation time: 30 minutes
Cooking time: 15 minutes
Serving: 4

Ingredients

- 2 tablespoons cream cheese or a mixture of 1 tablespoon cream cheese and 1 1/2 tablespoons shredded mozzarella cheese
- 1/2 tbsp of unsalted butter, melted
- 1 tablespoon finely shredded and chopped carrot
- 1 tablespoon of sweetener of your choice
- 1 tablespoon almond flour
- 1 teaspoon pumpkin pie spice
- 1/2 teaspoon keto friendly flavour of choice
- 1/2 teaspoon baking powder
- I pinch of salt
- 1 egg
- cream CHEESE FROSTING
- 1 tablespoon cream cheese
- 1tbsp unsalted butter
- 1 teaspoon sweetener of choice

Directions:

1. Making the cream CHEESE FROSTING

2. Heat the butter and cream cheese for the frosting

3. Mix until smooth and add the sweetener.

4. Making the chaffles

5. Heat up waffle maker.

6. Melt cheese cream, mozzarella, and butter for 15 seconds in a low heat

7. Mix flour, sweetener, flavour, salt

8. Mix the melted butter content with the dry ingredients

9. Whisk egg thoroughly

10. Gently whisk egg into the existing batter thoroughly

11. Add the carrot and the pumpkin pie spice. Mix thoroughly

12. Grease the waffle maker

13. Add batter to waffle maker

14. Repeat baking procedures till batter is finished

15. Drizzle the frosting over chaffles as desired.

27.Chocolate Chaffles with Raspberries

Preparation time: 5 minutes
Cooking time: 5 minutes
Serving: 4

Ingredients

- 2 cups almond/ coconut flour
- 1 tbsp. mozzarella cheese
- 2 tsps. baking powder
- Pinch of salt
- oz. unsweetened chocolate, coarsely chopped
- 1 ¾ cups Lekanto sugar free maple syrup
- 2 large eggs
- tbsps. unsalted butter, melted

- ½ pint fresh raspberries
- Berry Syrup
- 3 fresh berries
- 1 tsp. grated lemon zest
- ½ cup sweetener
- 1 tbsp. lemon juice

Directions:

1. Making the Berry Syrup

2. Mix the berries and ½ cup water in a large saucepan and boil over medium-high heat.

3. Crush the berries with the spoon or masher. Lower the heat and cook the mixture for 10 minutes.

4. Place a fine mesh sieve over a bowl or cup.

5. Pour the berries into the sieve, pressing lightly to release the juices.

6. Pour the juice in a small size saucepan and gently stir in the lemon zest, sugar and lemon juice. Boil over medium heat, stirring continuously to dissolve the sugar. Leave to simmer for about 8-10 minutes until the syrup has thickened slightly.

7. Serve warm or refrigerate for about 1 week

8. Making the Chaffles

9. Heat up a waffle iron.

10. In a bowl preferably large one, mix the flour, sweetener, baking powder and salt.

11. Stir in the chocolate.

12. Whisk the cheese, eggs and butter together in a separate medium bowl.

13. Gently mix the egg mixture into the dry ingredients.

14. Lightly grease the waffle iron.

15. Ladle the batter into the waffle iron.

16. Bake until crispy and golden brown, according to manufacturer's directions.

17. Repeat the baking procedure until all batter is baked.

18. Sprinkle with raspberries to serve.

19. Serve with berry syrup

20. Enjoy!

28. Yeast-Risen Overnight Chaffles

Preparation time: 10 minutes
Cooking time: 10 minutes
Servings: 4

Ingredients:

- 2 cups almond flour
- 1 tablespoon sweetener
- ½ teaspoon salt
- ½ teaspoon instant yeast
- 2 cups cheese, slightly warmed
- ½ cup unsalted butter, melt down and cooled to room temperature
- 1 teaspoon pure vanilla extract
- 2 large eggs, separated the next day

NOTE:

Warming the cheese gives the yeast a head start. Do not make it too hot or the yeast will die and the batter won't bubble.

Some versions of overnight waffles require the mixture to stay on the counter at room temperature.

Directions:

1. Mix the flour, sweetener, salt, and yeast in a large bowl.

2. In a medium-size bowl, Mix the cheese, butter, and vanilla together.

3. Gently mix the wet ingredients with

the dry ingredients.

4. Stir the mixture thoroughly.

5. Close up the mix with plastic wrap or a tight-fitting lid and leave for an hour at room temperature before refrigerating overnight.

6. The next morning, the batter will bubble a bit.

7. Preheat the waffle iron on medium Gently grease the waffle iron.

8. Preheat the oven on its lowest setting.

9. Stir the egg yolks into the batter.

10. Place the egg whites in a medium-size bowl, and beat them thoroughly.

11. Gently mix the dry and wet ingredients together until smooth.

12. Ladle the batter in the waffle iron and bake for about 3 to 5 minutes until light golden brown.

13. Bake all batter

14. Serve with butter and maple syrup.

29. Cocoa Chaffles with Coffee Cream recipe

Preparation time: 15 minutes
Cooking time: 15 minutes
Serving: 6

Ingredients:

- ½ cup heavy cream
- 1 tsp. espresso powder (or substitute 3 tbsps. espresso or strong brewed coffee)
- 2 tbsps. low carb sweetener of choice (Lekanto or monkfruit)
- 6 oz. mascarpone
- 2 cups almond flour
- 1 tbsp. baking powder
- 1 tsp. baking soda
- ¼ tsp. salt
- 1 tbsp. Dutch-process cocoa powder
- 3 large eggs
- 1 ¾ cups shredded mozzarella cheese
- 6 tbsps. Unsalted butter, melted
- 1/3 cup cacao nibs
- Dark chocolate shavings for garnish (optional)

Directions:

1. Making coffee cream:

2. In a medium bowl, mix the cream, espresso powder and 2 tbsps. of low carb sweetener of choice.

3. Whisk the cream thoroughly.

4. Fold in the mascarpone and set aside.

5. Making the chaffles:

6. Preheat a Waffle maker.

7. In a large bowl, mix the almond flour, baking powder, baking soda, salt and cocoa powder together

8. In a bowl preferably small size, whip the egg yolks till beaten, add the shredded cheese and melted butter together.

9. Create a hole in the dry ingredients, pour in the egg mixture, stir in the cacao nibs and mix to form a smooth batter.

10. Grease the waffle maker.

11. Ladle the batter in to the waffle maker, in 1/2 -3/4 cup measures.

12. Bake for about 3-4 minutes till chaffle is crispy and golden brown.

13. Take it out using a spatula and leave to cool. Repeat the baking process till the whole batter is finished.

14. Serve with coffee cream and sprinkle with chocolate shavings as desired.

15. Enjoy!

30. White mushroom chaffles with Salted Caramel Sauce

Preparation time: 15 minutes
Cooking time: 15 minutes
Servings: 4-6

Ingredients:

- 4 White mushrooms (washed and shredded)
- ¾ cup whole cheese
- 3 large eggs
- 4 tbsps. unsalted butter, melted
- 2 cups almond flour
- 2 tbsps. sweetener
- 1 ½ tbsps. baking powder
- ½ tsp. salt
- For 1 cup Salted Caramel Sauce
- ¼ cup sweetener
- 4 tbsps. unsalted butter, melted
- 1 tsp. vanilla
- ¾ cup cheese cream
- 1 tsp. salt

Directions:

1. Heat a Waffle iron beforehand according to manufacturer's instructions.
2. In a bowl (medium size), whisk the white mushroom, cheese, eggs and butter.
3. In a bowl (large size), mix the flour, brown sweetener, baking powder and salt together.
4. Gently mix the butter mixture into the dry ingredients until thoroughly mixed.
5. Lightly grease the waffle iron.

6. Ladle the batter in the preheated Waffle iron.
7. Bake until golden brown.
8. Repeat the baking procedure until all batter is baked.
9. Drizzle with the warm salted caramel to serve.

31. Lemon–Poppy seed chaffles

Preparation time: 10 minutes
Cooking time: 20 minutes
Serving: 6

Ingredients:

- 2 large eggs
- 11/2 cups cream cheese
- 1/2 cup (4 oz/125 g) no salt butter, melted
- 2 tablespoons finely grated lemon zest
- 2 tablespoons fresh lemon juice
- 1 teaspoon French vanilla flavor
- 11/2 cups (71/2 oz/235 g) almond flour
- 1/3 cup (3 oz/90 g) monk fruit or any keto-friendly sweetener of choice
- 11/2 teaspoons baking powder
- 1 teaspoon baking soda
- 1/4 teaspoon salt
- 2 tablespoons poppy seeds

Directions:

1. Making chaffle:
2. Heat a waffle maker beforehand
3. In a bowl (medium), whisk together the eggs, cheese, butter, lemon zest, lemon juice, and vanilla.
4. In a bowl (large), combine the flour, sweetener, baking powder, baking soda, and salt. Stir in the poppy seeds.

5. Create a hole in the center of the bowl containing the dry ingredients. Pour in the egg mixture.

6. Whisk thoroughly until mostly smooth.

7. Grease the waffle maker

8. Ladle the batter in the waffle maker, using 1/2–3/4 cup of batter per batch.

9. Bake for about 3-4 minutes until the waffles are crisp and golden brown.

10. Remove the waffles from the waffle maker.

11. Either you serve immediately or leave to cool before serving.

12. Top with the any keto-friendly sauce and dust with cheese.

32.Gingerbread Chaffles with sugar free maple syrup

Preparation time: 15 minutes
Cooking time: 15 minutes
Serving: 6

Ingredients:

- For the Maple Butter
- 6 tablespoons (3 oz/90 g) unsalted butter, softened
- 11/2 tablespoons pure maple syrup
- Pinch of salt
- Pinch of cinnamon
- For Chaffles
- 2 large eggs
- 11/2 cups of any keto cheese
- 1/2 cup (4 oz/125 g) no salt butter, melted,
- 1 teaspoon keto-friendly flavour of choice
- 11/2 cups (71/2 oz/235 g) almond/coconut flour

- 3 tablespoons Lekanto sugar free maple syrup
- 1 tablespoon baking powder
- 1 ½ teaspoons ground ginger
- 1 teaspoon cinnamon
- 1/4 teaspoon ground cloves

Directions:

1. Making maple butter:

2. To prepare the maple butter, in a bowl (small size) , whisk together the butter, maple syrup, cinnamon and salt. Scoop into a ramekin or other serving dish. Place it in the freezer for 5 minutes or in the refrigerator for 15 minutes to firm up before serving.

3. Making coffee cream:

4. Preheat a waffle maker

5. Whisk together the eggs, cheese, butter, and flavour in a medium bowl.

6. Mix the flour, sweetener, baking powder, ginger, cinnamon, cloves, and salt together in a large bowl.

7. Carefully pour the egg mixture into the dry ingredients.

8. Whisk thoroughly till smooth.

9. Grease the waffle maker

10. Ladle the batter into the waffle maker.

11. Cook for about 3-4 minutes till the waffles are crisp and browned.

12. Remove the waffles from the waffle maker and serve right away, or allow to cool before serving.

13. Top with pats of maple butter and/or drizzle with maple syrup

33.Peanut Butter and Jam (Peanut butter and Jam) chaffle

Preparation time: 15 minutes
Cooking time: 15 minutes

Serving: 6

Ingredients:

- For the Maple Butter
- 1 cup jam or preserves of your choice, such as raspberry, strawberry, or blackberry
- 2 large eggs
- 11/2 cups cheese of your choice
- ½ cup natural peanut butter
- 1/4 cup unsalted butter, melted,
- 11/2 cups (almond flour
- 3 tablespoons keto-friendly sweetener
- 1 tablespoon baking powder
- 1/2 teaspoon salt

Directions:

1. Making the jam
2. Place the jam in a small saucepan.
3. Heat for about 1 to 3 minutes until just gently warmed and loose enough to pour, stir continuously.
4. Stir and place in a serving bowl or pitcher.
5. Making chaffles
6. Preheat a waffle maker
7. Whip the eggs, milk, 1/2 cup peanut butter, and butter on medium speed for about 2 minutes in the bowl until smooth.
8. In a bowl (medium), mix together the flour, sugar, baking powder, and salt.
9. Add the dry ingredients to the peanut butter mixture until well mixed. Ladle the batter into the waffle maker.
10. Cook for about 3-4 minutes until the waffles are crisp and browned.
11. Remove the waffles from the waffle maker.
12. Repeat coking procedure until all batter if finished.
13. Cut chaffles into half, or quarters.
14. Place a waffle piece on a plate; spread some peanut butter on top.
15. Pour some of the warmed jam on top, then top with another piece of chaffle, or leave open-faced if desired.
16. Repeat with the remaining chaffles and serve right away or allow to cool.
17. Note: For best results, use salted but unsweetened peanut butter.

34. Cheddar Thyme Chaffles with Bacon Syrup

Preparation time: 15 minutes
Cooking time: 15 minutes
Serving: 4-6

Ingredients:

- For the cheddar thyme
- 2 cups almond/chocolate flour
- 2 tsps. baking powder
- 1 tsp. salt
- 2 large eggs
- 2 cups cream cheese
- tbsps. unsalted butter, melted
- 2 cups shredded cheddar
- 1 tsp. chopped fresh thyme
- 1 cup Bacon Syrup
- 1 lb. bacon, cut crosswise into 1" pieces
- 2 tsps. unsalted butter
- 3 tbsps. finely chopped onion
- ¼ cup desired sweetener
- 1 cup sugar free maple syrup

- 1 tsp. chopped fresh thyme
- ½ tsp. finely ground black pepper
- 1 tbsp. peanut oil

Directions:

1. Making the chaffles
2. Heat up the Waffle iron beforehand according to manufacturer's instructions.
3. Mix the flour, baking powder and salt in a large bowl.
4. Whip the eggs together in a separate medium bowl. Whisk in the cream cheese and melted butter until thoroughly mixed. Stir the butter mixture and cheddar cheese into the flour mixture until thoroughly mixed.
5. Grease the waffle maker.
6. Ladle the batter in the preheated waffle iron.
7. Bake until golden brown, according to manufacturer's directions.
8. Repeat baking procedure till batter is finished.
9. Serve with warm Bacon Syrup.
10. Making the bacon syrup
11. Line a large baking sheet with 2 layers of paper towels and set aside.
12. Add the bacon to a large skillet and heat on a low heat.
13. Cook the bacon for about 12-15 minutes, turn if needed, until the fat is rendered and the bacon is lightly browned all over, about 12–15 minutes.
14. Transfer the bacon to drain. Allow to cool slightly.
15. Finely chop bacon till crumbled. Set aside.
16. Pour off all but about 1 tbsp. of the bacon fat from the pan. Melt butter and heat for about 1 minute and add to the bacon fat. Add the onion to the pan and cook over medium heat. Stir continuously for about 7–10 minutes until translucent.
17. Add ½ cup water, maple syrup, thyme and black pepper, and bring to boil. Lower to a simmer and cook for 2 minutes, stirring and scraping up any browned bits. Add the bacon and mix well.
18. Cook uncovered for about 5–7 minutes, always stirring, until the liquid is slightly reduced and thickened.
19. Remove from the heat and stir in a little peanut oil. Serve warm or refrigerate for up to 1 week.

35. Chaffled Chicken Breast Stuffed with Spinach, Pine Nuts, and Feta

Preparation time:20 minutes
Cooking time: 15 minutes
Serving: 4-6

Ingredients

1. 1 cup finely chopped fresh baby spinach
2. 3/4 cup feta cheese, crumbled
3. 2 tablespoons toasted pine nuts
4. 2 cloves garlic, minced
5. ½ teaspoon dried thyme
6. 4 boneless, skinless chicken breast halves
7. ½ teaspoon salt
8. ½ teaspoon freshly ground black pepper

NOTE: The Use of baby spinach reduces the stress of picking through to remove large stems.

The use of toasted pine nut is to bring out the

flavor.

Directions:

1. Toasting the pine nut
2. Put the pine nuts inside a dry pan over medium heat.
3. Stir frequently till the nuts become fragrant and are barely turning brown.
4. Remove from the heat and pour them onto a plate to cool.
5. Making the Chaffles
6. Preheat the waffle iron and oven on medium.
7. Put the spinach, cheese, nuts, garlic, and thyme in a small bowl.
8. Smash together until the filling becomes cohesive and easier to handle.
9. Lightly grease the waffle iron
10. Make a parallel cut into the thickest portion of each chicken breast half to form a pocket. But do not to cut through.
11. Divide the combination into four equal parts and fill up each pocket in the chicken breasts, leaving a margin at the edge to close.
12. Season the chicken with salt and pepper.
13. Arrange the chicken into the waffle iron to allow lid to press down on the chicken more evenly.
14. Close the lid.
15. Cook the chicken for 8 minutes. Check and rotate if need be and cook for about 3 minutes. The chicken should be golden brown.
16. 6 Remove the chicken from the waffle iron
17. Repeat baking procedure with any remaining chicken.
18. Keep cooked chicken warm and serve warm.

36.Rich & Creamy Chaffles Recipe

Preparation time: 5 minutes
Cooking time: 5 minutes
Servings: 4-6

Ingredients

- 2 eggs
- 1 cup shredded mozzarella
- 2 tablespoons almond flour
- 2 tablespoons cream cheese
- 3/4 teaspoon baking power
- I pinch of salt
- 3 tablespoons water (optional)

Directions:

1. Making the Chaffles
2. Heat up the waffle iron on medium.
3. Mix cream cheese, egg, cheese, mozzarella in a small bowl.
4. Whisk egg thoroughly
5. Mix flour, baking powder, salt together in a large bowl
6. Gently whisk the egg mixture into the dry ingredients.
7. Whisk thoroughly until smooth
8. Lightly grease the waffle iron
9. Ladle the batter into the waffle maker
10. Bake till golden brown.
11. Repeat baking procedure till batter is finished.
12. Serve warm.

37.Light & Crispy Bacon Cheddar Chaffles Recipe

Preparation time: 5 minutes
Cooking time: 5 minutes
Servings: 4

Ingredients

- 2 egg
- 1 cup cheddar
- ½ Coconut/almond flour
- 1/2 teaspoon baking powder
- Bacon
- Shredded parmesan cheese on top and bottom.

Directions:

1. Making the Chaffles
2. Heat up the waffle iron on medium.
3. Mix eggs, cheddar cheese in a small bowl.
4. Whisk egg thoroughly
5. Mix flour, baking powder, salt together in a large bowl
6. Gently whisk the egg mixture into the dry ingredients.
7. Whisk thoroughly until smooth
8. Add the bacon into the mixture and mix thoroughly
9. Lightly grease the waffle iron
10. Ladle the batter into the waffle maker
11. Bake till crispy and golden brown.
12. Repeat baking procedure till batter is finished.
13. Serve warm.

38. Stuffed Chaffles

Preparation time: 15 minutes
Cooking time: 15 minutes
Servings: 6

Ingredients:

- 1 tablespoon extra-virgin olive oil
- 1/4 cup chopped onion
- ½ cup chopped celery
- ¾ teaspoon salt ½ teaspoon freshly ground black pepper
- ½ teaspoon poultry seasoning
- ¼ teaspoon dried sage
- 6 cups low-carb dry bread cubes (about ½-inch square)
- ½ cup unsalted butter, melted
- 1 cup low-sodium chicken broth
- 1 cup cheese
- 4 eggs (separated)

NOTE: Cut any slightly stale pieces or ends into cubes and leave at room temperature for an hour before using.

Directions:

1. Put the bread cubes in a bowl preferably big size.
2. Mix butter, cheese, egg white and chicken broth together in a medium bowl
3. In another bowl, mix all vegetables together
4. Pour the butter mixture over the bread.
5. Add the vegetable mixture and stir.
6. Leave the stuffing mixture to sit for 5 minutes to completely absorb the liquid, stir it once or twice.
7. Preheat the waffle iron on medium heat.
8. Lightly grease the waffle iron.
9. Put close to 1/2 cup of the stuffing mix on one section of the waffle iron.
10. Use enough of the mixture to slightly overstuff each section of the waffle iron.

11. Close the lid and press down to compress the stuffing.

12. Bake till golden brown and cohesive.

13. Repeat the baking procedure until all stuffing mixtures are baked.

14. Keep completed stuffles warm

15. Serve cool

39. Broccoli & Cheese Chaffle

Preparation Time: 5 minutes
Cooking Time: 8 minutes
Servings: 2

Ingredients:

- ¼ cup broccoli florets
- 1 egg, beaten
- 1 tablespoon almond flour
- ¼ teaspoon garlic powder
- ½ cup cheddar cheese

Directions:

1. Preheat your waffle maker.

2. Add the broccoli to the food processor.

3. Pulse until chopped.

4. Add to a bowl.

5. Stir in the egg and the rest of the ingredients.

6. Mix well.

7. Pour half of the batter to the waffle maker.

8. Cover and cook for 4 minutes.

9. Repeat procedure to make the next chaffle.

40. Chaffle with Sausage Gravy

Preparation Time: 5 minutes
Cooking Time: 15 minutes
Servings: 2

Ingredients:

- ¼ cup sausage, cooked
- 3 tablespoons chicken broth
- 2 teaspoons cream cheese
- 2 tablespoons heavy whipping cream
- ¼ teaspoon garlic powder
- Pepper to taste
- 2 basic chaffles

Directions:

1. Add the sausage, broth, cream cheese, cream, garlic powder and pepper to a pan over medium heat.

2. Bring to a boil and then reduce heat.

3. Simmer for 10 minutes or until the sauce has thickened.

4. Pour the gravy on top of the basic chaffles

5. Serve.

41. Crispy Keto Chaffle Bags

Preparation time: 30 minutes
Cooking time: 10 minutes
Servings: 14

Ingredients

- 90g stevia erythritol (sweetness 1: 1 like sugar)
- pieces of sweetener tabs (sweetness per tab 6g sugar)
- 100g almond flour
- 250ml unsweetened almond milk (I use alpro)
- 15g locust bean gum
- drops of vanilla flavor
- Melt 70g butter
- 5g coconut flour
- 40g protein powder vanilla (I use

sportness from DM)

- 15g egg white powder

Directions:

1. Finely grind the stevia erythritol and sweetener tabs. Stir the sweet mix into the melted butter.

2. Stir in the almond milk with a whisk. Now mix in almond flour, coconut flour, egg white and egg white powder and vanilla flavor.

3. Finally, sift carob flour over it and quickly work into the mixture.

4. Let the chaffle batter rest for about 10 minutes. In the meantime, preheat the croissant machine at the highest level.

5. Now reduce the temperature a little and place 1 to 1.5 tablespoons of the chaffle batter in the middle of the hot plate and spread lightly. Carefully close the lid and wait briefly (approx. 20 seconds) until the mass "bakes on" something.

6. Now push the lid all the way down, so that the dough spreads even further. After about 1 to 1 1/2 minutes, carefully remove the chaffle with a spatula from the croissant machine and place it on a worktop lined with baking paper.

7. Wait a moment - be careful, the chaffle is hot! After half a minute at the latest, place the chaffle over the chaffle cone and roll the cone gently back and forth and press the chaffle onto the overlapping ends. Let the chaffle cool down on the cone (it only takes so long until the next chaffle is baked, i.e. at the most 2 minutes.)

8. Bake more chaffles with the rest of the dough and either form a croissant (with a cone) or chaffle cups by pouring the hot chaffle over an upturned coffee cup and pressing it

down all around.

9. Let chaffles cool and serve either with ice cream or any other filling as desired.

10. If you like, you can refine the wafers with chocolate - either dip the top / bottom ends in chocolate and sprinkle with coconut flakes or grated nuts, or brush the chaffle cups with melted chocolate.

11. This brings an additional taste kick and prevents soaking

42. Pumpkin Keto Protein Pumpkin Vanilla

Preparation time: 30 minutes
Cooking time: 10 minutes
Servings: 6

Ingredients

- 1 egg
- 1 tablespoon of vanilla erithrite, passed through a sieve
- 1 pinch of cinnamon
- 15 grams of almond flour, passed through a sieve
- 1 teaspoon of baking soda
- 120 grams of mozzarella, grated
- 50 grams of Hokkaido pumpkin, grated

Directions:

1. Prepare the chaffle maker and switch it on so that it can preheat

2. In a small bowl, whisk the egg with the vanilla and cinnamon.

3. Gradually add baking soda and almond flour. I always sift it into the mix because I only work with the whisk. The recipe is so easy and there is no need to get any equipment dirty.

4. Now add the mozzarella to the egg-flour mixture and stir with a fork until the cheese is well covered.

5. Finally, stir in the pumpkin.

6. Bake the chaffles in 2 portions over medium heat. The recipe makes 2 chaffles for my heart chaffle maker. The dough does not stick anywhere in me even without fat, even with lean mozzarella.

7. You should consume the finished chaffles immediately. For this reason, I personally make only half the recipe when my husband is not at home. You can't taste the cheese directly hot from the iron - I don't think my husband even suspects that I could make an omelets filled with grated pumpkin and cheese.

8. When warming up in the microwave or in the toaster, a slight taste of cheese reappears.

9. So maybe cut the recipe in half! Fresh tastes best.

43. Keto Protein Chaffles

Preparation time: 40 minutes
Cooking time: 15 minutes
Servings: 11

Ingredients

- 5 pieces size M eggs
- 100 grams of pea protein I take this because it has low carbohydrates: pea protein
- 100 grams of cream
- 3 grams of baking powder
- 30 grams of butter
- 100 grams of mineral water
- 60 grams of almond cream
- 75 grams of stevia erythritol I'll take

this: erythritol + stevia
- 15 grams of Amaretto Aroma

Preparation

1. Separate egg white and egg yolk.

2. Put all ingredients except the egg white in the bowl and stir.

3. Keto-protein chaffles-2

4. Beat the egg white into egg whites and fold in carefully.

5. Bake the chaffles in the chaffle iron. (Makes 11 chaffles in this chaffle iron size)

44. Basic Recipe For Cheese Chaffles

Preparation time: 40 minutes
Cooking time: 15 minutes
Servings: 2

Ingredients

- 1 medium or large egg
- 50 g of grated mozzarella (fresh, self-grated is less suitable) cheesebutter
- Salt
- Pepper

Directions:

1. While the chaffle iron is heating, whisk the egg and then fold in the fresh mozzarella.

2. Season with pepper and salt and add a little butter to the iron. As soon as it is melted and well distributed, add the dough and bake the cheese chaffles until they are golden brown and crispy. Salty chaffles of this type taste both warm and cold.

45. Prepare Hearty Chaffle Dough With Jalapeno

Preparation time: 10 minutes

Cooking time: 5 minutes
Servings: 2

Ingredients

- 3 large eggs
- 2 to 3 jalapenos, cored, one diced, the other cut into strips
- 4 slices of bacon
- 225 g cream cheese
- 115 g grated cheddar cheese
- 3 tbsp coconut flour
- 1 teaspoon Baking powder
- 1/4 tsp Himalayan salt

Directions:

1. Fry the bacon until crispy in a pan. In the meantime, mix the dry ingredients together and beat the cream cheese in a separate bowl until creamy. Heat the chaffle iron and grease it. Whisk the eggs and fold in half of the cream cheese and cheese, then the dry ingredients. Finally, fold in the diced jalapenos.

2. Bake the cheese wafers by putting half of the dough in the iron, taking out the chaffle after about 5 minutes and then baking the other half.

3. Serve the chaffles with the rest of the cream cheese, the bacon and the remaining jalapenos.

47.Cheese Chaffle Recipe With Cinnamon, Vanilla & Almond Flour

Preparation time: 10 minutes
Cooking time: 5 minutes
Servings: 2

Ingredients

- 1 egg
- 115 g grated mozzarella

- 1 tbsp almond flour
- 1 teaspoon Baking powder
- 1 tsp vanilla extract
- 1 pinch of cinnamon Fat for the chaffle maker

Directions:

1. Mix the egg with the vanilla extract. Mix the dry ingredients in a separate bowl and add them to the egg. Finally, fold in the cheese, grease the chaffle iron and pour half of the dough into it. Now bake the chaffle for about 5 minutes or until it is golden brown and crispy. Check periodically so that it doesn't burn. Repeat with the other half of the batter and serve the still warm chaffles with a little butter and low-carb syrup as you like.

47.Keto Chocolate Twinkie Copycat Chaffle

Preparation time: 5 minutes
Cooking time: 12 minutes
Servings: 3

Ingredients

- 2 tablespoons of butter (cooled)
- 2 oz cream cheese softened
- Two large egg room temperature
- 1 teaspoon of vanilla essence
- 1/4 cup Lacanto confectionery
- Pinch of pink salt
- 1/4 cup almond flour
- 2 tablespoons coconut powder
- 2 tablespoons cocoa powder
- 1 teaspoon baking powder

Directions:

2. Preheat the Maker of Corndog.

3. Melt the butter for a minute and let it cool.

4. In the butter, whisk the eggs until smooth.

5. Remove sugar, cinnamon, sweetener and blend well.

6. Add flour of almond, flour of coconut, powder of cacao and baking powder.

7. Blend until well embedded.

8. Fill each well with ~2 tablespoons of batter and spread evenly.

9. Close the lid and let it cook for 4 minutes.

10. Lift from the rack and cool it down.

48.Keto Blueberry Chaffle

Preparation time: 5 minutes
Cooking time: 15 minutes
Servings: 5

Ingredients

- 1 cup mozzarella cheese
- 2 tablespoons almond flour
- 1 tsp baking powder
- 2 eggs
- 1 tsp cinnamon
- Sweetner 2 tsp
- 3 tablespoons blueberry

Directions:

1. Heat up your waffle maker Dash mini.

2. Place mozzarella cheese, almond flour, baking powder, milk, cinnamon, and blueberries in a mixing bowl. Blend well in order to blend all the ingredients together.

3. Spray the non-stick cooking spray on your mini waffle maker.

4. Attach a cup of blueberry keto waffle

batter in a little less than 1/4.

5. Close the lid and cook 3-5 minutes of the chaffle. Check to see if it's crispy and golden at the 3-minute mark. If it is not or if it sticks to the top of the waffle cooker, close the lid and cook for 1-2 more minutes.

6. Serve with a drop of sugar or keto syrup from swerve confectioners.

7. Notes Net carbs-2 g net carbs per chaffle of blueberry

49.Easy Corndog Chaffle Recipe

Preparation time: 10 minutes
Cooking time: 4 minutes
Servings: 5

Ingredients:

- 2 eggs
- 1 cup Mexican cheese blend
- 1 tbs almond flour
- 1/2 tsp cornbread extract
- 1/4 tsp salt
- hot dogs with hot dog sticks

Directions:

1. Preheat corndog waffle maker.

2. In a small bowl, whip the eggs.

3. Add the remaining ingredients except the hotdogs

4. Spray the corndog waffle maker with non-stick cooking spray.

5. Fill the corndog waffle maker with the batter halfway filled.

6. Place a stick in the hot dog.

7. Place the hot dog in the batter and slightly press down.

8. Spread a small amount of better on top of the hot dog, just enough to fill it.

9. Makes about 4 to 5 chaffle corndogs

10. Cook the corndog chaffles for about 4 minutes or until golden brown.

11. When done, they will easily remove from the corndog waffle maker with a pair of tongs.

12. Serve with mustard, mayo, or sugar-free ketchup!

50.Krispy Kreme Copycat of Glazed Raspberry Jelly-Filled Donut

Preparation time: 10 minutes
Cooking time: 3 minutes

Ingredients:

- 1 egg
- 1/4 cup mozzarella cheese shredded
- 2 T cream cheese softened
- 1 T sweetener
- 1 T almond flour
- 1/2 tsp Baking Powder
- 20 drops glazed donut flavoring
- Raspberry Jelly Filling Ingredients:
- 1/4 cup raspberries
- 1 tsp chia seeds
- 1 tsp confectioners sweetener
- Donut Glaze Ingredients
- 1 tsp powdered sweetener
- A few drops of water or heavy whipping cream

Instructions:

Directions:

1. Mix everything together to make the chaffles first.

2. Cook for about 2 1/2-3 minutes.

3. Make the Raspberry Jelly Filling:

4. Mix together in a small pot on medium heat.

5. Gently mash raspberries.

6. Let cool.

7. Add between the layers of Chaffles.

8. Make the Donut Glaze:

9. Stir together in a small dish.

10. Drizzle on top Chaffle.

51.Rice Krispie Treat Chaffle Copycat Recipe

Preparation time: 15 minutes
Cooking time: 5 minutes
Servings: 2

Ingredients:

- Chaffle batter:
- 1 Large Egg room temp
- 2 oz. Cream Cheese softened
- 1/4 tsp Pure Vanilla Extract
- 2 tbs Lakanto Confectioners Sweetener
- 1 oz. Pork Rinds crushed
- 1 tsp Baking Powder
- Marshmallow Frosting:
- 1/4 c. Heavy Whipping Cream
- 1/4 tsp Pure Vanilla Extract
- 1 tbs Lakanto Confectioners Sweetener
- 1/2 tsp Xanthan Gum

Directions:

1. Plug in the mini waffle maker to preheat.

2. In a medium mixing bowl- Add egg, cream cheese, and vanilla.

3. Whisk until blended well.

4. Add sweetener, crushed pork rinds,

and baking powder.

5. Mix until well incorporated.

6. Sprinkle extra crushed pork rinds onto waffle maker (optional).

7. Then add about 1/4 scoop of batter over, sprinkle a bit more pork rinds.

8. Cook 3-4 minutes, then remove and cool on a wire rack.

9. Repeat for remaining batter.

10. Make the Marshmallow Frosting:

11. Whip the HWC, vanilla, and confectioners until thick and fluffy.

12. Slowly sprinkle over the xanthan gum and fold until well incorporated.

13. Spread frosting over chaffles and cut as desired, then refrigerate until set.

14. Enjoy cold or warm slightly in the microwave for 10 seconds.

52. Biscuits & Gravy Chaffle Recipe

Preparation time: 10 minutes
Cooking time: 5 minutes
Servings: 4

Ingredients:

- 2 tbs Unsalted Butter melted
- 2 Large Eggs
- 1 c. Mozzarella Cheese shredded
- 1 tbs Garlic minced
- drops Cornbread Extract optional
- 1/2 tbs Lakanto Confectioners optional
- 1 tbs Almond Flour
- 1/4 tsp Granulated Onion
- 1/4 tsp Granulated Garlic
- 1 tsp Dried Parsley
- 1 tsp Baking Powder

- 1 batch Keto Sausage Biscuits and Gravy Recipe

Directions:

1. Preheat Mini Waffle Maker.

2. Melt the butter, let cool.

3. Whisk in the eggs, then fold in the shredded cheese.

4. Add the rest of ingredients and mix thoroughly.

5. Scoop 1/4 of batter onto waffle maker and cook 4 minutes.

6. Remove and let cool on wire rack.

7. Repeat for the remaining 3 chaffles.

53. Keto Tuna Melt Chaffle Recipe

Preparation time: 15 minutes
Cooking time: 8 minutes
Servings: 2

Ingredients:

- 1 packet Tuna 2.6 oz with no water
- 1/2 cup mozzarella cheese
- 1 egg
- pinch salt

Directions:

1. Preheat the mini waffle maker

2. In a small bowl, add the egg and whip it up.

3. Add the tuna, cheese, and salt and mix well.

4. Optional step for an extra crispy crust: Add a teaspoon of cheese to the mini waffle maker for about 30 seconds before adding the recipe mixture. This will allow the cheese to get crispy when the tuna chaffle is done cooking. I prefer this method!

5. Add 1/2 the mixture to the waffle maker and cook it for a minimum of 4

minutes.

6. Remove it and cook the last tuna chaffle for another 4 minutes.

54.Blueberry & Brie Grilled Cheese Chaffle

Preparation time: 10 minutes
Cooking time: 10 minutes

Ingredients:

- 2 Chaffles
- 1 T Blueberry Compote
- 1 oz Wisconsin Brie sliced thin
- 1 T Kerrygold butter
- Chaffle Ingredients:
- 1 egg, beaten
- 1/4 cup mozzarella shredded
- 1 tsp Swerve confectioners
- 1 T cream cheese softened
- 1/4 tsp baking powder
- 1/2 tsp vanilla extract
- Blueberry Compote Ingredients:
- 1 cup blueberries washed
- Zest of 1/2 lemon
- 1 T lemon juice freshly squeezed
- 1 T Swerve Confectioners
- 1/8 tsp xanthan gum
- 2 T water

Directions:

1. Mix everything together.
2. Cook 1/2 batter for 2 1/2- 3 minutes in the mini waffle maker
3. Repeat.
4. Let cool slightly on a cooling rack.
5. Blueberry Compote Instructions:

6. Add everything except xanthan gum to a small saucepan. Bring to a boil, reduce heat and simmer for 5-10 minutes until it starts to thicken. Sprinkle with xanthan gum and stir well.
7. Remove from heat and let cool. Store in refrigerator until ready to use.
8. Grilled Cheese Instructions:
9. Heat butter in a small pan over medium heat. Place Brie slices on a Chaffle and top with generous 1 T scoop of prepared blueberry compote.
10. Place sandwich in pan and grill, flipping once until waffle is golden and cheese has melted, about 2 minutes per side.

55.BBQ Chicken Chaffle

Preparation time: 3 minutes
Cooking time: 8 minutes
Servings: 2

Ingredients:

- 1/3 cup cooked chicken diced
- 1/2 cup shredded cheddar cheese
- 1 tbsp sugar-free bbq sauce
- 1 egg
- 1 tbsp almond flour

Directions:

1. Heat up your Dash mini waffle maker.
2. In a small bowl, mix the egg, almond flour, BBQ sauce, diced chicken, and Cheddar Cheese.
3. Add 1/2 of the batter into your mini waffle maker and cook for 4 minutes. If they are still a bit uncooked, leave it cooking for another 2 minutes. Then cook the rest of the batter to make a second chaffle.
4. Do not open the waffle maker before

the 4 minute mark.

5. Enjoy alone or dip in BBQ Sauce or ranch dressing!

56.Cheddar Chicken and Broccoli Chaffle

Preparation time: 2 minutes
Cooking time: 8 minutes
Servings: 2

Ingredients:

- 1/4 cup cooked diced chicken
- 1/4 cup fresh broccoli chopped
- Shredded Cheddar cheese
- 1 egg
- 1/4 tsp garlic powder

Directions:

1. Heat up your Dash mini waffle maker.
2. In a small bowl, mix the egg, garlic powder, and cheddar cheese.
3. Add the broccoli and chicken and mix well.
4. Add 1/2 of the batter into your mini waffle maker and cook for 4 minutes. If they are still a bit uncooked, leave it cooking for another 2 minutes. Then cook the rest of the batter to make a second chaffle and then cook the third chaffle.
5. After cooking, remove from the pan and let sit for 2 minutes.
6. Dip in ranch dressing, sour cream, or enjoy alone.

57.Spinach & Artichoke Chicken Chaffle

Preparation time: 3 minutes
Cooking time: 8 minutes
Servings: 2

Ingredients:

- 1/3 cup cooked diced chicken
- 1/3 cup cooked spinach chopped
- 1/3 cup marinated artichokes chopped
- 1/3 cup shredded mozzarella cheese
- 1 ounce softened cream cheese
- 1/4 teaspoon garlic powder
- 1 egg

Directions:

1. Heat up your Dash mini waffle maker.
2. In a small bowl, mix the egg, garlic powder, cream cheese, and Mozzarella Cheese.
3. Add the spinach, artichoke, and chicken and mix well.
4. Add 1/3 of the batter into your mini waffle maker and cook for 4 minutes. If they are still a bit uncooked, leave it cooking for another 2 minutes. Then cook the rest of the batter to make a second chaffle and then cook the third chaffle.
5. After cooking, remove from the pan and let sit for 2 minutes.
6. Dip in ranch dressing, sour cream, or enjoy alone.

58.Chicken Bacon Ranch Chaffle

Preparation time: 3 minutes
Cooking time: 8 minutes
Servings: 2

Ingredients:

- 1 egg
- 1/3 cup cooked chicken diced
- 1 piece bacon cooked and crumbled
- 1/3 cup shredded cheddar jack cheese

- 1 teaspoon powdered ranch dressing

Directions:

1. Heat up your Dash mini waffle maker.

2. In a small bowl, mix the egg, ranch dressing, and Monterey Jack Cheese.

3. Add the bacon and chicken and mix well.

4. Add half of the batter into your mini waffle maker and cook for 3-4 minutes. Then cook the rest of the batter to make a second chaffle.

5. Remove from the pan and let sit for 2 minutes.

6. Dip in ranch dressing, sour cream, or enjoy alone.

59. Buffalo Chicken Chaffle Recipe

Preparation time: 10 minutes
Cooking time: 5 minutes
Servings: 6

Ingredients:

- 1 Can Valley Fresh Organic Canned Chicken Breast (5 ounces)
- 2 T Red Hot Wing Sauce
- 2 oz Cream Cheese softened
- 4 T Cheddar Cheese shredded
- 2 T Almond Flour
- 1 T Nutritional Yeast
- 1/2 tsp Baking Powder
- 1 Egg Yolk Can Use whole egg if no allergy
- 1 Flax Egg 1 T ground flaxseed, 3 T water
- 1/4-1/2 Cup Extra Cheese for the waffle iron

Directions:

1. Make flax egg and set aside to rest.

2. Drain liquid from the canned chicken. Mix all the ingredients together. Sprinkle a little cheese on the waffle iron. Let it sit for a few seconds before adding 3 T of chicken mixture — Cook for 5 minutes.

3. Don't open the waffle iron before the time is up, or you will have a mess. Remove and let cool before adding a drizzle of hot sauce and ranch dressing.

Note:

The whole recipe is 6.4 carbs. Each Chaffle is 1.1 carb.

60. Jamaican Jerk Chicken Chaffle

Preparation time: 5 minutes
Cooking time: 10 minutes
Servings: 4

Ingredients:

- Jamaican Jerk Chicken Filling:
- 1 pound organic ground chicken browned or roasted leftover chicken finely chopped
- 2 tablespoons Kerrygold butter
- 1/2 medium onion chopped
- 1 teaspoon granulated garlic
- 1 teaspoon dried thyme
- 1/8 teaspoon black pepper
- 2 teaspoon dried parsley
- 1 teaspoon salt
- 2 teaspoon Walker's Wood Jerk Seasoning Hot and Spicy jar type paste
- 1/2 cup chicken broth
- Chaffle Ingredients:
- 1/2 cup mozzarella cheese
- 1 tablespoon butter melted

- 1 egg well beaten
- 2 tablespoon almond flour
- 1/4 teaspoon baking powder
- 1/4 teaspoon turmeric
- A pinch of xanthan gum
- A pinch of salt
- A pinch of garlic powder
- A pinch of onion powder

Directions:

1. In a medium saucepan, cook onion in the butter.
2. Add all spices and herbs. Saute until fragrant.
3. Add chicken.
4. Stir in chicken broth.
5. Cook on low for 10 minutes.
6. Raise temperature to medium-high and reduce liquid until none is left in the bottom of the pan.
7. Enjoy!

61.Wasabi Chaffles

Preparation time: 15 minutes
Cooking time: 15 minutes
Servings: 1

Chaffle Ingredients:

- Classic Chaffle Recipe
- Japanese Toppings Ingredients:
- 1 whole avocado, ripe
- 5 slices of pickled ginger
- 1 tbsp of gluten-free soy sauce
- 1/3 of a cup of edamame
- 1/4 of a cup of Japanese pickled vegetables
- 1/2 pound of sushi-grade salmon,

sliced
- 1/4 of a tsp of wasabi
- Tools: waffle maker, mini or regular sized, one mixing bowl, measuring cups and tablespoons, spatula, non-stick cooking spray (or butter), blender, electric beaters, or whisk.

Directions:

1. Cut the salmon and avocado into thin slices. Set aside.
2. If the edamame is frozen, boil it in a pot of water until done. Set aside.
3. Follow the Classic Chaffle recipe.
4. Once the chaffles are done, pour a tablespoon of soy sauce onto the chaffle and then layer the salmon, avocado, edamame, pickled ginger, pickled vegetables, and wasabi.
5. Enjoy!

62.Loaded Chaffle Nachos

Preparation time: 15 minutes
Cooking time: 15 minutes
Servings: 1

Chaffle Ingredients:

- Classic Chaffle Recipe
- Nacho Ingredients:
- Taco Meat recipe
- 1 whole avocado, ripe
- 1/2 cup of sour cream
- 1/2 of a cup of cheddar cheese, shredded
- 1/2 an onion
- 1 handful of cilantro, chopped
- 1 lime, cut into wedges
- hot sauce of your choice
- Tools: waffle maker, mini or regular

40

sized, one mixing bowl, measuring cups and tablespoons, spatula, non-stick cooking spray (or butter), blender, electric beaters, or whisk.

Directions:

1. Dice the cilantro, lettuce, onions, and limes.

2. Shred the cheese in a bowl. Melt if desired.

3. Follow instructions for the Taco Meat recipe.

4. Follow the Classic Chaffle recipe.

5. Once the chaffles are done, rip them into triangles.

6. Spread the chaffle triangles onto a plate and layer on the sour cream, meat, avocado, onions, cilantro, cheese, and lime.

7. Enjoy!

63.Mozzarella Panini

Preparation time: 15 minutes
Cooking time: 15 minutes
Servings: 1

Chaffle Ingredients:

- Classic Chaffle Recipe
- Sandwich Filling Ingredients:
- 1 ounce of mozzarella, thinly sliced
- 1 heirloom tomato, thinly sliced
- 1/4 of a cup of pesto
- 2 fresh basil leaves
- Tools: waffle maker, mini or regular sized, one mixing bowl, measuring cups and tablespoons, spatula, non-stick cooking spray (or butter), blender, electric beaters, or whisk.

Directions:

1. Follow the Classic Chaffle recipe.

2. Once the chaffles are done, lay two side by side.

3. Spread the pesto on one, then layer the mozzarella cheese and tomatoes and sandwich together.

64.Lox Bagel Chaffle

Preparation time: 15 minutes
Cooking time: 15 minutes
Servings: 1

Chaffle Ingredients:

- Classic Chaffle Recipe or Sweet Chaffle Recipe
- 2 tbsps of Everything Bagel Seasoning
- Filling Ingredients:
- 1 ounce of cream cheese
- 1 beefsteak tomato, thinly sliced
- 4-6 ounces of salmon gravlax
- 1 small shallot, thinly sliced
- capers
- 1 tbsp of fresh dill
- Tools: waffle maker, mini or regular sized, one mixing bowl, measuring cups and tablespoons, spatula, non-stick cooking spray (or butter), blender, electric beaters, or whisk.

Directions:

1. Slice the tomato and the shallots.

2. Follow the Classic Chaffle recipe and add the everything bagel seasoning.

3. Once the chaffles are done, sprinkle more everything bagel seasoning onto the tops of both chaffles.

4. Lay two chaffles side by side and layer on the cream cheese, salmon, and shallots.

5. Sprinkle dill and capers and sandwich the two chaffles together.

6. Enjoy!

65. Cuban Sandwich Chaffle

Preparation time: 15 minutes
Cooking time: 15 minutes
Servings: 1

Chaffle Ingredients:

- Classic Chaffle Recipe
- Cubano Ingredients:
- 1/4 of a pound of ham, cooked and sliced
- 1/4 of a pound of pork, roasted and sliced
- 1/4-pound Swiss cheese, thinly sliced
- 3 dill pickles, sliced in half
- Tools: waffle maker, mini or regular sized, three mixing bowls, measuring cups and tablespoons, spatula, non-stick cooking spray (or butter), baking sheet, blender, electric beaters, or whisk.

Directions:

1. Follow the Classic Chaffle recipe.
2. Take two chaffles and lay side by side.
3. Lay on the meat, cheese, and pickles.
4. Sandwich the two chaffles together.
5. Put the sandwich in a toaster oven if you want it hot.
6. Heat for 5 minutes or until cheese is melted.

66. Parmesan garlic chaffles

Preparation time: 10 minutes
Cooking time: 5 minutes

Ingredients

- 1/2 cup shredded mozzarella cheese
- 1 whole egg, beaten
- 1/4 cup grated Parmesan cheese
- 1 teaspoon Italian Seasoning
- 1/4 teaspoon garlic powder

Directions

1. Start pre-heating your waffle maker, and let's start preparing the batter.
2. Add in all the ingredients, except for the mozzarella cheese to a bowl and whisk. Add in the cheese and mix until well combined.
3. Spray your waffle plates with nonstick spray and add half the batter to the center. Close the lid and cook for 3-5 minutes, depending on how crispy you want your Chaffles.
4. Serve with a drizzle of olive oil, grated Parmesan cheese and fresh chopped parsley or basil.

67. Key lime Chaffle

Preparation time: 10 minutes
Cooking time: 5 minutes

Ingredients (for 3 to 4 mini chaffles)

Chaffle ingredients

- 1 egg
- 2 tsp cream cheese room temp
- 1 tsp powdered sweetener swerve or monkfruit
- 1/2 tsp baking powder
- 1/2 tsp lime zest
- 1/4 cup Almond flour
- 1/2 tsp lime extract or 1 tsp fresh squeezed lime juice
- Pinch of salt

Cream Cheese Lime Frosting ingredients

- 4 oz cream cheese softened

- 4 tbs butter
- 2 tsp powdered sweetener swerve or monkfruit
- 1 tsp lime extract
- 1/2 tsp lime zest

Directions:

1. Preheat the mini waffle iron.
2. In a blender add all the chaffle ingredients and blend on high until the mixture is smooth and creamy.
3. Cook each chaffle about 3 to 4 minutes until it's golden brown.
4. While the chaffles are cooking, prepare the frosting.
5. In a small bowl, combine all the ingredients for the frosting and mix until smooth.
6. Allow the chaffles to completely cool before frosting them.

68. Jicama Loaded Baked Potato Chaffle

Preparation time: 10 minutes
Cooking time: 15 minutes

Ingredients

- 1 cup cheese of choice
- 2 eggs, whisked
- 1 large jicama root
- 1/2 medium onion, minced
- Salt and Pepper
- 2 garlic cloves, pressed

Directions:

1. Peel jicama and shred in food processor
2. In a large colander, place the shredded jicama, and sprinkle with 1-2 tsp of salt. Mix well and allow to drain.
3. Squeeze out as much liquid as possible.
4. Microwave for 5-8 minutes
5. Mix all ingredients together
6. Sprinkle a little cheese on waffle iron, then add 1/3 of the mixture, and sprinkle a little more cheese on top of the mixture.
7. Cook for 5 minutes. Flip and cook 2 more.
8. Top with a dollop of sour cream, bacon pieces, cheese, and chives.

69. Chaffle Mcgriddles

Preparation time: 10 minutes
Cooking time: 5 minutes

Ingredients

- 1 Egg
- 3/4 cup Shredded Mozzarella
- 1 Sausage Patty
- 1 Slice American Cheese
- 1 tbsp Sugar-Free Flavored Maple Syrup
- 1 tbsp Swerve or Monkfruit (or any sugar replacement of choice)

Directions:

- Pre-heat your Mini Waffle Maker
- Beat the egg into a small mixing bowl,
- Add shredded Mozzaerlla, Swerve/Monkfruit, Maple Syrup and mix until well combined.
- Place ~2 tbsp of the resulting egg mix onto the Dash Mini Waffle Maker, close lid and cook for 3 – 4 minutes. Repeat for as many waffles you are making.
- Meanwhile, follow cooking

instructions for sausage patty and place cheese onto patty while still warm to melt.

- Assemble Chaffle McGriddle and enjoy!

70.Light & Crispy Chaffles

Preparation time: 10 minutes
Cooking time: 5 minutes

Ingredients

- 1 egg
- 1/3 cup cheddar
- 1/4 teaspoon baking powder
- 1/2 teaspoon ground flaxseed
- Shredded parmesan cheese on top and bottom.

Directions:

1. Mix the ingredients together and cook in a mini waffle iron for 4-5 minutes until crispy.

2. Once cool, enjoy your light and crisp Keto waffle.

3. You can experiment with seasonings to the initial mixture depending on the mood of your taste buds.

71.Chaffle Sandwich With Bacon And Egg

Preparation time: 10 minutes
Cooking time: 5 minutes

Ingredients

- 1 large egg
- 1/2 cup of shredded cheese
- thick-cut bacon
- fried egg
- sliced cheese

Instructions

1. Preheat your waffle maker.

2. In a small mixing bowl, mix together egg and shredded cheese. Stir until well combined.

3. Pour one half of the waffle batter into the waffle maker. Cook for 3-4 minutes or until golden brown. Repeat with the second half of the batter.

4. In a large pan over medium heat, cook the bacon until crispy.

5. In the same skillet, in 1 tbsp of reserved bacon drippings, fry the egg over medium heat. Cook until desired doneness.

6. Assemble the sandwich, and enjoy!

72.Rich Creamy Chaffles

Preparation time: 5 minutes
Cooking time: 5 minutes
Servings: 4

Ingredients:

- 1 egg
- ½ cup mozzarella cheese, shredded
- Oil of grease
- Heavy crème
- Salt & pepper to taste

Directions:

1. Heat the waffle maker. Take a bowl add egg or mozzarella cheese and whisk all together. Add some salt or pepper as per taste and mix all together. Spray the oil to grease the waffle maker. Now pour the mixture into the maker and cook for 4 minutes or until golden brown. Repeat the process for the whole batter. Serve the chaffle with heavy crème layer.

73.Bacon & Cheddar Cheese Chaffles

Preparation time: 5 minutes
Cooking time: 5 minutes
Servings: 6

Ingredients:

- ½ cup almond flour
- 3 bacon strips
- ¼ cup sour cream
- 1 ½ cup cheddar cheese
- ½ cup smoked Gouda cheese
- ½ tsp onion powder
- ½ tsp. baking powder
- ¼ cup oat
- 1 egg
- 1 tbsp. oil
- 1 ½ tbsp. butter
- ¼ tsp. salt
- ½ tsp. parsley
- ¼ tsp. baking soda

Directions:

1. Heat the waffle maker. Take a bowl add almond flour, baking powder, baking soda, onion powder, garlic salt and mix well. In another bowl whisk eggs, bacon, cream, parsley, butter and cheese until well combined. Now pour the mixture over dry ingredients and mix well. Pour the batter over the preheated waffle maker and cook for 5 to 6 minutes or until golden brown. Serve the hot and crispy chaffles.

74.Jalapeno & Bacon Chaffle

Preparation time: 5 minutes
Cooking time: 5 minutes
Servings: 6

Ingredients:

- 3 tbsp. coconut flour

- 1 tsp baking powder
- 3 eggs
- 8 oz. cream cheese
- ¼ tsp salt
- 4 bacon slices
- 2 to 3 jalapeno
- 1 cup cheddar cheese

Directions:

1. Wash the jalapeno and slice them. Take a pan and cook jalapeno until golden brown or crispy. Take a bowl add flour, baking powder and salt and mix. In a mixing bowl add cream and beat well until fluffy. Now in another bowl add egg and whisk them well. Pour cream, cheese and beat until well combine. Add the mixture with dry ingredients and make a smooth batter. After that fold the jalapeno in prepare mixture. Heat the waffle maker and pour the batter into it. Cook it for 5 minutes or until golden brown. Top it with cheese, jalapeno and crème and serve the hot chaffles.

75.Light & Crispy Bagel Chaffle Chips

Preparation time: 5 minutes
Cooking time: 5 minutes
Servings: 4

Ingredients:

- 3 tbsp. parmesan cheese
- 1 tsp oil for grease
- 1 tsp bagel seasoning
- Salt and pepper to taste

Directions:

1. Preheat the waffle maker. Add the parmesan cheese in the pan and melt it well. Now pour the melted

parmesan cheese over the waffle maker and sprinkle bagel seasoning over the cheese. Cook the mixture for about 2 to 3 minutes without closing the lid. Let it settle or turn crispy for 2 minutes then remove and serve the crispy chis crunch.

76.Coconut Flour Waffle

Preparation time: 5 minutes
Cooking time: 5 minutes
Another Chaffle you can prepare is the Coconut flour waffle.

Ingredients

- 8 eggs
- 1/2 cup of butter or coconut oil (melted)
- 1 tsp of vanilla extract
- 1/2 tsp salt
- 1/2 cup of coconut flour

Directions

1. Pre heat the mini waffle maker,
2. Whisk the eggs in a bowl,
3. Then you add the melted butter or coconut oil, cinnamon, vanilla and salt, mix properly then you add the Coconut flour.
4. Ensure the batter is thick,
5. Add the mixture into the mini waffle maker and allow to cook till it has a light brown appearance.
6. Serve with butter or maple syrup.

77.Cream Cheese Waffle

Preparation time: 10 minutes
Cooking time: 5 minutes
You can make your own Cream Cheese Waffles and serve them with Honey Whipped Cream for breakfast

Ingredients

- 2 cups of flour
- 1 tsp baking powder
- 1/8 tsp salt
- 2 tsp light brown sugar
- 4 ounces of 1/3 Less Fat Cream Cheese ,
- 2 eggs
- 1/2 cups of milk
- 2 tablespoons canola oil
- 1/2 tablespoon pure vanilla extract
- 4 tablespoons honey

Directions

1. First step is to preheat the mini waffle maker.
2. Then you mix the flour, baking powder, salt and light brown sugar; mix thoroughly to ensure uniformity.
3. In your bowl, add the cream cheese and egg yolks; mix until smooth.
4. Then you Add milk, oil and vanilla; mix properly.
5. Add flour mixture to cream cheese mixture and stir until moist. Set
6. The next step is to Place egg whites in a bowl and beat until it forms a stiff peak.
7. Using a spatula, fold the egg whites gently into the waffle-batter; fold just until thoroughly combined.
8. Pour 1/3-cup of the batter onto the preheated mini waffle iron.
9. Allow to cook for about 2 to 3 minutes, or until it has a light brown appearance
10. Next step is to prepare the Whipped Cream.Pour the heavy cream into a large mixing bowl and beat on until it

becomes thick.

11. Add honey and continue to beat until soft peaks form. When ready,

12. Serve waffles topped with Honey Whipped Cream and fresh berries (if you prefer).

78.. Keto Taco Chaffle

Preparation time: 10 minutes
Cooking time: 4 minutes
Love tacos? You can prepare your own special keto Taco Chaffle.

Ingredients

- 1/2 cup cheese (cheddar or mozzarella), shredded
- 1 egg
- 1/4 teaspoon Italian seasoning
- Taco Meat seasoning for ground beef
- You have to prepare your Taco meat separately, you'll need the following ingredients for Taco meat seasoning;
- 1/4 cup chili powder
- 1/4 cup ground cumin
- 2 tablespoons garlic powder
- 2 tablespoons cocoa powder
- 1 tablespoon onion powder
- 1 tablespoon salt
- 1 teaspoon smoked paprika

Directions

1. You have to Cook your ground beef or ground turkey first Separately. Add all the taco meat seasonings.

2. While making the taco meat, start making the keto chaffles.

3. First step is to Pre-heat the mini waffle maker.

4. Whisk the egg in a small bowl,

5. Add the shredded cheese and seasoning.

6. Place half the chaffle mixture into the mini waffle maker and allow it to cook for about 3 to 4minutes.

7. Repeat and cook the second half of the mixture to make the second chaffle.

8. Add the warm taco meat to your taco chaffle. You can Top it with lettuce, tomatoes, cheese, and serve.

79.Brownie Chaffle

Preparation time: 5 minutes
Cooking time: 3 minutes
If you love brownies, then you should try this brownie Chaffle recipe which is very easy to make and is ready in few minutes.

Ingredients

- 1 Egg Whisked
- 1/3 cup Mozzarella Cheese Shredded
- 1 ½ tbsp Cocoa Powder Dutch Processed
- 1 tbsp Almond Flour
- 1 tbsp Monkfruit Sweetener
- 1/4 tsp Vanilla extract
- 1/4 tsp Baking Powder
- Pinch of Salt
- 2 tsp Heavy Cream

Directions

1. First step as always is to preheat your mini waffle iron.

2. Next, whisk the egg. Add the dry ingredients. Then add the cheese in a bowl. Then you Pour 1/3 of the batter on the waffle iron. Allow to cook for 3 minutes or until steam stops coming out of the waffle iron.

3. Serve with your favorite low carb toppings.

80.White Bread Keto Chaffle

Preparation time: 5 minutes
Cooking time: 4 minutes
This is similar to a traditional Chaffle, but it is more of a regular bread than a Chaffle.

Ingredients

- 2 egg whites
- cream cheese, melted
- 2 tsp water
- 1/4 tsp baking powder
- 1/4 cup almond flour
- 1 Pinch of salt

Directions

1. Pre-heat the mini waffle maker,

2. Whisk the egg whites together with the cream cheese and water in a bowl.

3. Next step is to add the baking powder, almond flour and salt and whisk until you have a smooth batter. Then you pour half of the batter into the mini waffle maker.

4. Allow to cook for roughly 4 minutes or until you no longer see steam coming from the waffle maker.

5. Remove and allow to cool.

81. Cranberry and Brie Chaffle

Preparation time: 10 minutes
Cooking time: 20 minutes
Servings: 4 mini chaffles

Ingredients:

- 4 tablespoons frozen cranberries
- 3 tablespoons swerve sweetener
- 1 cup / 115 grams shredded brie cheese
- 2 eggs, at room temperature

Directions:

1. Take a non-stick waffle iron, plug it in, select the medium or medium-high heat setting and let it preheat until ready to use; it could also be indicated with an indicator light changing its color.

2. Meanwhile, prepare the batter and for this, take a heatproof bowl, add cheese in it, and microwave at high heat setting for 15 seconds or until cheese has softened.

3. Then add sweetener, berries, and egg into the cheese and whisk with an electric mixer until smooth.

4. Use a ladle to pour one-fourth of the prepared batter into the heated waffle iron in a spiral direction, starting from the edges, then shut the lid and cook for 4 minutes or more until solid and nicely browned; the cooked waffle will look like a cake.

5. When done, transfer chaffles to a plate with a silicone spatula and repeat with the remaining batter.

6. Let chaffles stand for some time until crispy and serve straight away.

82.Banana Foster Chaffle

Preparation time: 10 minutes
Cooking time: 20 minutes
Servings: 4 large chaffles

Ingredients:

- For Chaffle:
- 1/8 teaspoon cinnamon
- ½ teaspoon banana extract, unsweetened
- 4 teaspoons swerve sweetener
- 1 cup / 225 grams cream cheese, softened
- ½ teaspoon vanilla extract,

unsweetened

- 8 eggs, at room temperature
- For Syrup:
- 20 drops of banana extract, unsweetened
- 8 teaspoons swerve sweetener
- 20 drops of caramel extract, unsweetened
- drops of rum extract, unsweetened
- 8 tablespoons unsalted butter
- 1/8 teaspoon cinnamon

Directions:

1. Take a non-stick waffle iron, plug it in, select the medium or medium-high heat setting and let it preheat until ready to use; it could also be indicated with an indicator light changing its color.

2. Meanwhile, prepare the batter for chaffle and for this, take a large bowl, crack eggs in it, add sweetener, cream cheese, and all the extracts and then mix with an electric mixer until smooth, let the batter stand for 5 minutes.

3. Use a ladle to pour one-fourth of the prepared batter into the heated waffle iron in a spiral direction, starting from the edges, then shut the lid and cook for 5 minutes or more until solid and nicely browned; the cooked waffle will look like a cake.

4. When done, transfer chaffles to a plate with a silicone spatula, repeat with the remaining batter and let chaffles stand for some time until crispy.

5. Meanwhile, prepare the syrup and for this, take a small heatproof bowl, add butter in it, and microwave at high heat setting for 15 seconds until it melts.

6. Then add remaining ingredients for the syrup and mix until combined.

7. Drizzle syrup over chaffles and then serve.

83.Flaxseed Chaffle

Preparation time: 10 minutes
Cooking time: 20 minutes
Servings: 4 medium chaffles

Ingredients:

- 2 cups ground flaxseed
- 2 teaspoons ground cinnamon
- 1 teaspoon of sea salt
- 1 tablespoon baking powder
- 1/3 cup / 80 ml avocado oil
- 5 eggs, at room temperature
- ½ cup / 120 ml water
- Whipped cream as needed for topping

Directions:

1. Take a non-stick waffle iron, plug it in, select the medium or medium-high heat setting and let it preheat until ready to use; it could also be indicated with an indicator light changing its color.

2. Meanwhile, prepare the batter and for this, take a large bowl and then stir in flaxseed, salt and baking powder until combined.

3. Crack the eggs in a jug, pour in oil and water, whisk these ingredients until blended and then stir this mixture into the flour with the spatula until incorporated and fluffy mixture comes together.

4. Let the batter stand for 5 minutes and then stir in cinnamon until mixed.

5. Use a ladle to pour one-fourth of the prepared batter into the heated waffle

iron in a spiral direction, starting from the edges, then shut the lid and cook for 5 minutes or more until solid and nicely browned; the cooked waffle will look like a cake.

6. When done, transfer chaffle to a plate with a silicone spatula and repeat with the remaining batter.

7. Top waffles with whipped cream and then serve straight away.

84. Hazelnut Chaffle

Preparation time: 10 minutes
Cooking time: 30 minutes
Servings: 6 mini chaffles

Ingredients:

- 1 cup / 100 grams hazelnut flour
- ½ teaspoon baking powder
- 2 tablespoons hazelnut oil
- 1 cup / 245 grams almond milk, unsweetened
- 3 eggs, at room temperature

Directions:

1. Take a non-stick waffle iron, plug it in, select the medium or medium-high heat setting and let it preheat until ready to use; it could also be indicated with an indicator light changing its color.

2. Meanwhile, prepare the batter and for this, take a large bowl, add flour in it, stir in the baking powder until mixed and then mix in oil, milk, and egg with an electric mixer until smooth.

3. Use a ladle to pour one-sixth of the prepared batter into the heated waffle iron in a spiral direction, starting from the edges, then shut the lid and cook for 5 minutes or more until solid and nicely browned; the cooked waffle will look like a cake.

4. When done, transfer chaffle to a plate with a silicone spatula and repeat with the remaining batter.

5. Let chaffles stand for some time until crispy and serve straight away.

85. Maple Pumpkin Chaffle

Preparation time: 5 minutes
Cooking time: 4 minutes
Servings: 2

Ingredients:

- 2 eggs
- 3/4 tsp baking powder
- 2 tsp 100% pumpkin puree
- 3/4 tsp pumpkin pie spice
- 4 tsp heavy whipping cream
- 2 tsp sugar-free maple syrup
- 1 tsp coconut flour
- 1/2 cup mozzarella cheese, shredded
- 1/2 tsp vanilla
- Pinch of salt

Directions:

1. Preheat the waffle maker.

2. Combine all ingredients in a small mixing bowl.

3. If you're using a mini waffle maker, pour around 1/4 of the batter. Allow to cook for 3-4 minutes.

4. Repeat.

86. Nutty Chaffles

Preparation time: 5 minutes
Cooking time: 5 minutes
Servings: 1

Ingredients:

- 1 egg

- 1 tsp coconut flour
- 1 1/2 tbsp unsweetened cocoa
- 2 tbsp sugar-free sweetener
- 1 tbsp heavy cream
- 1/2 tsp baking powder
- 1/2 tsp vanilla

Directions:

1. Preheat the waffle maker.

2. Combine all the ingredients in a small bowl. Mix well.

3. Pour half the batter into the waffle maker. Allow to cook for 3-5 minutes until golden brown and crispy.

4. Carefully remove and add the remaining batter.

87.Crispy Chaffle With Everything But The Bagel Seasoning

Preparation time: 5 minutes
Cooking time: 5 minutes
Servings: 1

Ingredients:

- 2 eggs
- 1/2 cup parmesan cheese
- 1 tsp everything but the bagel seasoning
- 1/2 cup mozzarella cheese
- 2 tsp almond flour

Directions:

1. Preheat the waffle maker.

2. Sprinkle the mozzarella cheese onto the waffle maker. Let it melt and cook for 30 seconds until crispy. Remove this from the waffle maker.

3. Using a whisk, combine eggs, parmesan, almond flour, seasoning, and the toasted cheese in a small bowl.

4. Pour the batter into the waffle maker.

5. Allow the batter to cook for 3-4 minutes until crispy and golden brown in color.

88.Strawberry And Cream Cheese Low-Carb Keto Waffles

Preparation time: 5 minutes
Cooking time: 5 minutes
Servings: 2

Ingredients:

- 2 tsp coconut flour
- 4 tsp monkfruit
- 1/4 tsp baking powder
- 1 egg
- 1 oz cream cheese, softened
- 1/2 tsp vanilla extract
- 1/4 cup strawberries

Directions:

1. Preheat the waffle maker.

2. In a bowl put in the coconut flour, then add the baking powder and the monkfruit.

3. Add in the egg, cream cheese, and vanilla extract. Mix well with a whisk.

4. Pour the batter into the preheated waffle maker and allow to cook for 3-4 minutes.

5. Allow chaffles to cool before topping with strawberries.

89.Pumpkin Chaffle With Cream Cheese Glaze

Preparation time: 5 minutes
Cooking time: 5 minutes
Servings: 1

Ingredients:

- 1 egg
- 1/2 cup mozzarella cheese
- 1/2 tsp pumpkin pie spice
- 1 tbsp pumpkin
- For the cream cheese frosting:
- 2 tbsp cream cheese, softened at room temperature
- 2 tbsp monkfruit
- 1/2 tsp vanilla extract

Directions:

1. Preheat the waffle maker.
2. Whip the egg in a small bowl.
3. Add cheese, pumpkin, and pumpkin pie spice to the whipped egg and mix well.
4. Add half the batter to the waffle maker and allow to cook for 3-4 minutes.
5. While waiting for the chaffle to cook, combine all the ingredients for the frosting in another bowl. Continue mixing until a smooth and creamy consistency is reached. Feel free to add more butter if you prefer a more buttery taste.
6. Allow the chaffle to cool before frosting it with cream cheese.

90.Crunch Cereal Cake Chaffle

Preparation time: 10 minutes
Cooking time: 5 minutes

Servings: 1
(Does not include the toppings)

Ingredients:

- For the chaffles:
- 1 egg
- 2 tbsp almond flour
- 1/2 tsp coconut flour
- 1 tbsp butter, melted
- 1 tbsp cream cheese, softened
- 1/4 tsp vanilla extract
- 1/4 tsp baking powder
- 1 tbsp confectioners sweetener
- 1/8 tsp xanthan gum
- For the toppings:
- 20 drops captain cereal flavoring
- Whipped cream

Directions:

1. Preheat the mini waffle maker.
2. Blend or mix all the chaffles ingredients until the consistency is creamy and smooth. Allow to rest for a few minutes so that the flour absorbs the liquid ingredients.
3. Scoop out 2-3 tbsp of batter and put it into the waffle maker. Allow to cook for 2-3 minutes.
4. Top the cooked chaffles with freshly whipped cream.
5. Add syrup and drops of Captain Cereal flavoring for a great flavor.

SANDWICH CHAFFLES

91. Katsu Chaffle Sandwich

Preparation time: 90 minutes
Required cooking time: 22 minutes
Servings: 2

Ingredients:

- Sauce
- Ketchup: 2 tablespoons (sugar-free)
- Swerve/Monk fruit: 1 teaspoon
- Worcestershire Sauce: 2 tablespoons
- Oyster Sauce: 1 tablespoon
- Chaffle
- Green Leaf Lettuce: 2 leaves (optional)
- Egg: 2
- Mozzarella cheese: 1 cup (shredded)
- Chicken
- Chicken thigh: 2 pieces boneless or ¼ lb boneless
- Egg: 1
- Black pepper: ¼ teaspoon or as per your taste
- Vegetable oil: 2 cups (deep frying)
- Almond flour: 1 cup
- Salt: ¼ teaspoon or as per your taste
- Pork Rinds: 3 oz. unflavored
- Brine
- Water: 2 cups
- Salt: 1 tablespoon

Directions:

1. Using a skillet, boil the chicken with salt and 2 cups of water. With the lid closed, boil for 28 minutes. Once done, dry the chicken using a small towel to pat, then add salt and dried pepper on its sides. Using a mixing bowl, prepare a mixture containing the oyster sauce, monk fruit, sugar-free ketchup and Worcestershire and set aside. Using a food processor or blender, grind the pork rinds to fine crumbs. Using 3 mixing bowls containing the ingredients respectively (Almond flour, beaten eggs in another and the crushed pork in the last), coat the chicken using the ingredients in these bowls in this order (Flour-Eggs-Pork). Deep fry the chicken pieces in a frying pan to a golden brown, then place in a rack for excess oil to drip out.

2. Using another mixing bowl prepare a mix containing shredded mozzarella cheese with beaten eggs. With a closed lid, mix evenly and heat the waffle for 5 minutes to a crunch. Once timed out, remove the chaffle from the waffle maker. Repeat for the remaining chaffles mixture. Slice the avocados with the green leaf lettuce washed and dried. With one chaffle, spread sauce on it, the green lettuce, chicken katsu and close with another chaffle. Serve the dish and savour the taste.

92.Keto Sandwich Chaffle

Preparation time: 12 minutes
Required cooking time: 6 minutes
Servings: 2

Ingredients:

- Egg: 2
- Almond flour: 2 tablespoons
- Cheddar cheese: 1½ cup (shredded)

Directions:

1. Preheat and grease a waffle maker. Prepare a mixture containing cheddar cheese with beaten eggs, then mix evenly. Add the almond flavour to taste. Pour the evenly mixed batter into the waffle batter. With the lid closed, cook for 5 minutes to a crunch. Repeat the process for the remaining mixture. Once ready, garnish the chaffles in between as desired. Serve and enjoy.

93.Bread Sandwich Chaffle

Preparation time: 18 minutes
Required cooking time: 12 minutes
Servings: 2

Ingredients:

- Almond flour: 1 tablespoon
- Mayo: 2 tablespoon
- Garlic powder: ½ teaspoon
- Egg: 2
- Water: 2 teaspoon
- Baking powder: 1/8 teaspoon

Directions:

01. Prepare a mix of ingredients in a mixing bowl. Preheat and grease the waffle maker. Pour in the mixture into the waffle maker and spread evenly. Heat the mixture to a crispy form. Repeat the process to make as many chaffles as possible from the remaining.

94.Chaffle Sandwich With Eggs And Bacon

Preparation time: 12 minutes
Required cooking time: 6 minutes
Servings: 2

Ingredients:

- Sandwich
- Bacon strips: 4
- Egg: 2
- American cheese: 2 slices
- Chaffles
- Egg: 2
- Cheddar cheese: 1 cup (shredded)

Directions:

01. Preheat and grease the waffle maker. Using a mixing bowl prepare a mix containing shredded cheddar with beaten eggs. Blend to a froth, then add the earlier chocolate mixture. Mix evenly and pour into the lower side of the waffle maker. With a closed lid, heat the waffle for 5 minutes to a crunch and then remove the chaffle. Heat the sliced bacon to a crispy form using medium heat in a non-stick large pan, drain the fried bacon then fry the eggs. Put off the heat on the chaffle. Repeat for the remaining chaffles mixture to make more batter. Serve egg and cheese with slices of bacon in between two chaffles and enjoy.

95.Bbq Chicken Chaffle Sandwich

Preparation time: 1 hr
Cooking time: 30 mins

Ingredients:

- Boneless chicken breast 2 pieces
- BBQ Sauce (sugar-free)
- ¼ tsp paprika
- 1 tablespoon lime juice
- ¼ tsp of salt
- ¼ tsp of pepper
- 1 piece of coal

- ½ cup of cheddar cheese
- 1 egg
- ½ tablespoon of Italian herbs
- 1 slice of cheese
- ½ tomato (sliced)
- 2 slices of lettuce
- ½ tablespoon oil

Directions:

1. To make your BBQ chicken chaffle sandwich, start by the preparation of your chicken. Take the boneless chicken pieces and cut them into cubes.

2. Then marinate the cubes with Italian herbs, paprika, lime juice, oil, salt, and pepper. Then mix them thoroughly. Let the marination set on the chicken for around 20 minutes.

3. Then melt the butter in a pan and cook your chicken in it.

4. Take the piece of coal and burn it. Use a tong to pick it up and place it in an aluminum foil. Put the coal on the chicken and cover it with a lid.

5. Let the chicken cook with the smoky flavor for around 7 to 10 minutes.

6. Then remove the chicken and place it in a dish. Then start preparing your chaffle bread. Preparing the chaffle bread is easy and requires only two ingredients. Whisk together egg and cheddar cheese.

7. You can add some Italian seasonings to give some taste to the bread. Then preheat your waffle maker to medium heat and pour the mixture into the machine.

8. Cook it well for about 3 to 5 minutes. Repeat the process to get another chaffle.

9. Then assemble your sandwich. Put the chicken into the chaffle bread and add tomatoes, lettuce, bbq sauce, and a cheese slice to your sandwich. Voila! Your keto sandwich is ready.

Equipment:

Waffle machine

Pan

Bowl for marination

Aluminum foil

Nutrition:

Calories 388

Carbohydrates 2 g

Protein 21.1 g

Fat 18 g

96.Cajun Shrimp And Avocado Chaffle

Preparation time: 45 mins
Cooking time: 30 mins

Ingredients:

- 1 egg
- ½ cup of shredded cheddar cheese
- 1 tablespoon of almond flour
- 2 tsp of Cajun seasoning
- 1 lb raw shrimp
- 1 tablespoon of avocado oil
- 2 slices of bacon
- ⅓ cup of sliced red onions

Directions:

1. This sandwich is full of nutrients and contains a lot of ingredients. So let's start by preparing the ingredients. To begin with, heating a pan to medium heat with avocado oil. Then add the bacon strips to the pan and let each

side cook until crispy and brown.

2. Remove the bacon strips and dry them on a paper towel. This will help absorb excess oil.

3. Then prepare the shrimps. Put them in a bowl and add 1 tsp of Cajun seasoning. Add a small amount of avocado oil and salt and pepper. Leave them for 15 minutes.

4. Then put the shrimps in the pan and fry them in the same bacon grease. Fry each side for a small amount of time. Once they are fried, dry them on kitchen paper. Scoop out the avocado in a bowl.

5. Then prepare your chaffle bread. For the chaffle bread, add an egg with shredded cheddar cheese, almond flour, 1 tsp of cajun seasoning and cook in waffle machine that is preheated to medium heat for around 3 to 4 minutes.

6. Then assemble your Cajun Shrimp and Avocado chaffle sandwich. Add the shrimps, onions, bacon slices, and avocado. Then your scrumptious sandwich will be ready.

Equipment:

waffle maker

Pan

Bowl for marination

Nutrition:

Calories 390

Carbohydrates 2.5 g

Protein 19 g

Fat 16 g

97.Chickfila Like Chaffle Sandwich

Preparation time: 45 mins
Cooking time: 15 mins

Ingredients:

- 1 chicken breast
- 4 tablespoon of pickle juice
- 2 ½ tablespoon of cheddar cheese (powdered)
- 2 ½ tablespoon of pork rinds
- 1 tablespoon of flaxseed
- 2 tablespoon of melted butter
- ¼ tsp of salt
- ¼ tsp of pepper
- ½ tsp paprika
- 1 egg
- ½ cup of cheddar cheese (shredded)
- 2 slices of pickle

Directions:

1. For this recipe, you need to focus on preparing the chicken. Therefore, first of all, get your chicken and cut it into two pieces.

2. Keep these pieces in a zip lock bag with pickle juice. Make sure you let your chicken absorb the pickle juice for at least 2 hours to overnight for best taste.

3. Ensure that you keep the chicken in the refrigerator.

4. In a bowl, add dry ingredients such as pork rinds, flaxseed, powdered cheese, paprika, salt, and pepper.

5. Mix these ingredients. Prepare your air fryer. Preheat it to around 400 degrees.

6. Then take out the chicken and drain the pickle water. Dip the chicken in the unsalted butter and then into the mixture. Then let it cook in the air fryer from around 7 to 9 minutes.

7. Now prepare your chaffle keto bread. For the preparation of this low carb

bread, add an egg and shredded cheddar cheese to a bowl. Then beat the mixture and place it in a waffle machine that is preheated to medium heat for around 3 to 4 minutes.

8. After making your chaffle bread assembles the sandwich. Add chicken to the chaffle bread and top it off with cheese and pickle slices.

Equipment:

Airfryer

Waffle maker

Bowl

Nutrition:

Calories 525

Carbohydrates 2g

Protein 19 g

Fat 12 g

98.Salami Chaffle Sandwich

Preparation time:
Cooking time:

Ingredients:

- 2 Salami patties
- 2 tablespoon of coconut oil
- ¼ tsp of salt
- 1 slice of cheddar cheese
- 2 slices of lettuce
- 2 slices of tomato
- 1 egg
- ½ cup of mozzarella cheese (shredded)
- 1 tsp of Italian seasoning

Directions:

1. Start by the preparation of the salami patties. Take a pan and heat it to medium heat. Put 2 tablespoons of coconut oil in the pan and let it melt.

2. Then add your salami patties to the oil and let them fry.

3. Once they are fried, keep them on kitchen paper to absorb any excess oil.

4. Now you can prepare your chaffle bread. This bread can be prepared by adding an egg and shredded mozzarella cheese to a bowl.

5. Whisk these ingredients together and add Italian seasoning to give a spicy taste and pour the mixture in a waffle machine that is preheated to medium heat for around 3 to 4 minutes until the chaffle turns golden brown.

01. Now comes the part of the assembly of the sandwich. Add the salami, cheese slice, lettuce, and tomato to the chaffle bread.

Equipment:

Waffle maker

Pan

Bowl

Nutrition:

Calories 512

Carbohydrates 2.3 g

Protein 14 g

Fat 15 g

99.Reuben Chaffle Sandwich

Preparation time: 15 mins
Cooking time: 5 mins

Ingredients:

- 1 egg
- ½ cup of shredded cheddar cheese
- 1 tablespoon of almond flour

- 1 tablespoon of low carb thousand island sauce
- Pinch of baking powder
- 2 slices of corned beef
- 1 slice of mozzarella cheese
- 1 tablespoon sauerkraut

Directions:

1. Start by preparing your chaffle bread. The chaffle bread is a great low carb bread alternative.

2. All you need for this bread is an egg and shredded mozzarella cheese. Add them items along with baking powder, coconut flour, 1 tablespoon of thousand islands sauce in a bowl.

3. Whisk these ingredients together. Then preheat your waffle machine to around 450 degrees.

4. When it is warm enough, you should pour the mixture into the waffle machine. Let the chaffle cook for around 3 to 4 minutes until you see the golden brown color.

5. Once your chaffle bread is prepared, then start preparing your meet. Take a microwave-friendly plate and add the beef slice to it.

6. Top it off with the cheese slice and microwave it until the cheese melts.

7. Add the thousand island sauce and sauerkraut on the chaffle bread. Place your meat in the sandwich and enjoy.

Equipment:

Waffle Machine

Nutrition:

Serving size 1
Calories 490
Fat 21 g
Protein 16 g
Carbohydrates 3.1 g

100.Breakfast Chaffle Sandwich

Preparation time: 30 mins
Cooking time: 5 mins

Ingredients:

- 1 egg
- ½ cup of shredded mozzarella cheese
- 2 Tablespoon of coconut flour
- ½ tsp of baking powder
- 1 teaspoon of Italian herbs
- 2 tablespoon of almond oil
- 2 slices of tomato
- 2 slices of lettuce

Directions:

1. This is a simple breakfast chaffle that is very easy to cook and does not require a lot of ingredients. Begin by preparing the base of the chaffle.

2. You can do so by taking shredded mozzarella, egg, baking powder, and Italian herbs together in a bowl. Mix them well.

3. Then turn on your waffle machine to medium heat. Pour the batter in the waffle machine.

4. Don't open the machine before 3 minutes and let it cook until it is golden brown.

5. Now you can take a pan and turn on the heat to medium. Then add the unsalted butter in the pan and let it melt.

6. Once the butter melts, add chaffle and cook it in the butter until it becomes crispy.

7. Make sure you cook both sides well. Then assemble your sandwich. Add your vegetables in the sandwich and enjoy your healthy and nutritious breakfast.

Equipment:

Bowl

Waffle Machine

Pan

Nutrition:

Serving size 1
Calories 514
Fat 32g
Protein 22g
Carbohydrates 3g

101Bacon And Cheese Chaffle Sandwich

Preparation time: 30 mins
Cooking time: 5 mins

Ingredients:

- 1 egg
- ½ cup of shredded mozzarella cheese
- 2 Tablespoon of coconut flour
- ½ tsp of baking powder
- 1 teaspoon of Italian herbs
- 2 tablespoon of almond oil
- 1 slice of cheddar cheese
- 2 bacon strips

Directions:

1. The bacon and cheese chaffle sandwich is a great lunch or brunch food item. You can easily make this sandwich. It does not require any complicated ingredients.

2. Start with a simple chaffle base. Mix in a bowl shredded mozzarella cheese, coconut flour, baking powder, Italian herbs, and an egg.

3. Whisk this mixture well. Then take a waffle machine and preheat it to around medium heat.

4. Once it is preheated, sprinkle some cheese on the waffle machine. Add the mixture on top of the cheese base and top it off with more cheese.

5. Let this cook in the machine for 4 minutes until the color changes to a golden brown.

6. Then turn the heat below a pan. Then add almond oil in the pan, cook the bacon strips in the oil. Take them out once they are fried.

7. Now it is time for the assembly of the sandwich. Add your bacon and cheese to the sandwich and enjoy it.

Equipment:

Bowl

Waffle Machine

Pan

Nutrition:

Serving size 1
Calories 449
Fat 30g
Protein 24g
Carbohydrates 2.2g

102.Grilled Cheese Chaffle Sandwich

Preparation time: 45 mins
Cooking time: 10 mins

Ingredients:

- 1 egg
- ½ cup of cheddar cheese (shredded)
- ¼ teaspoon of baking powder
- ¼ tsp of garlic powder
- 2 slices of American cheese
- 1 ½ tablespoon of butter

Directions:

1. The best recipe is saved for the last! Who does not like themselves a grilled cheese sandwich? It is voted to be the best sandwich. Therefore, let's see how you can create a keto version of it. You will begin with the chaffle bread.

2. To make the chaffle bread. Begin your preparation by mixing in a bowl shredded cheddar cheese, baking powder, and the egg.

3. Once you have mixed them thoroughly, turn your waffle machine and preheat it to around medium heat. Once it is preheated, pour the mixture on the machine and close the lid.

4. The chaffle should cook for at least 3 to 4 minutes until the color changes to a golden brown. Repeat the process to have two chaffles.

5. Then take a pan and turn heat below it to medium. During that time, place two slices of your favorite cheese (in this case, American cheese) in between two chaffles. Put butter on the pan and allow it to melt.

6. Once the butter has melted, add a chaffle cheese sandwich to the pan and cook each side for at least 1 minute.

7. Remove the sandwich from the pan and enjoy your hot and tasty keto sandwich.

Equipment:

Pan

Waffle Maker

Bowl

Nutrition:

Calories 549
Carbohydrates 3g
Protein 27 g

Fat 48 g

103.Chaffle Cheese Sandwich

Preparation Time: 5 Min
Cooking Time: 10 Min
Servings: 1

Ingredients

- 2 square keto chaffle
- 2 slice cheddar cheese
- 2 lettuce leaves

Directions:

1. Prepare your oven on 4000 F.

2. Arrange lettuce leave and cheese slice between chaffles.

3. Bake in the preheated oven for about 4-5 minutes until cheese is melted.

4. Once the cheese is melted, remove from the oven.

5. Serve and enjoy!

104.Chaffle Egg Sandwich

Preparation Time: 5 Min
Cooking Time: 10 Min
Servings: 2

Ingredients

- 2 MINI keto chaffle
- 2 slice cheddar cheese
- 1 egg simple omelet

Directions:

1. Prepare your oven on 4000 F.

2. Arrange egg omelet and cheese slice between chaffles.

3. Bake in the preheated oven for about 4-5 minutes until cheese is melted.

4. Once the cheese is melted, remove from the oven.

5. Serve and enjoy!

105. Ham, Cheese & Tomato Chaffle Sandwich

Preparation Time: 5 minutes
Cooking Time: 10 minutes
Servings: 2

Ingredients:

- 1 teaspoon olive oil
- 2 slices ham
- 4 basic chaffles
- 1 tablespoon mayonnaise
- 2 slices Provolone cheese
- 1 tomato, sliced

Directions:

1. Add the olive oil to a pan over medium heat.
2. Cook the ham for 1 minute per side.
3. Spread the chaffles with mayonnaise.
4. Top with the ham, cheese and tomatoes.
5. Top with another chaffle to make a sandwich.

106. Creamy Chicken Chaffle Sandwich

Preparation Time: 5 minutes
Cooking Time: 10 minutes
Servings: 2

Ingredients:

Cooking spray

- 1 cup chicken breast fillet, cubed
- Salt and pepper to taste
- ¼ cup all-purpose cream
- 4 garlic chaffles
- Parsley, chopped

Directions:

1. Spray your pan with oil.
2. Put it over medium heat.
3. Add the chicken fillet cubes.
4. Season with salt and pepper.
5. Reduce heat and add the cream.
6. Spread chicken mixture on top of the chaffle.
7. Garnish with parsley and top with another chaffle.

107. Egg & Chives Chaffle Sandwich Roll

Preparation Time: 5 minutes
Cooking Time: 0 minute
Servings: 2

Ingredients:

- 2 tablespoons mayonnaise
- 1 hard-boiled egg, chopped
- 1 tablespoon chives, chopped
- 2 basic chaffles

Directions:

1. In a bowl, mix the mayo, egg and chives.
2. Spread the mixture on top of the chaffles.
3. Roll the chaffle.

108. Pulled Pork Chaffle Sandwiches

Preparation Time: 20 minutes
Cooking Time: 28 minutes
Servings: 4

Ingredients:

- 2 eggs, beaten
- 1 cup finely grated cheddar cheese

- ¼ tsp baking powder
- 2 cups cooked and shredded pork
- 1 tbsp sugar-free BBQ sauce
- 2 cups shredded coleslaw mix
- 2 tbsp apple cider vinegar
- ½ tsp salt
- ¼ cup ranch dressing

Directions:

1. Preheat the waffle iron.
2. In a medium bowl, mix the eggs, cheddar cheese, and baking powder.
3. Open the iron and add a quarter of the mixture. Close and cook until crispy, 7 minutes.
4. Transfer the chaffle to a plate and make 3 more chaffles in the same manner.
5. Meanwhile, in another medium bowl, mix the pulled pork with the BBQ sauce until well combined. Set aside.
6. Also, mix the coleslaw mix, apple cider vinegar, salt, and ranch dressing in another medium bowl.
7. When the chaffles are ready, on two pieces, divide the pork and then top with the ranch coleslaw. Cover with the remaining chaffles and insert mini skewers to secure the sandwiches.
8. Enjoy afterward.

109.Peanut Butter Sandwich Chaffle

Preparation Time: 15 minutes
Servings: 1

Ingredients:

- For chaffle:
- 1 egg, lightly beaten
- 1/2 cup mozzarella cheese, shredded

- 1/4 tsp espresso powder
- 1 tbsp unsweetened chocolate chips
- 1 tbsp Swerve
- 2 tbsp unsweetened cocoa powder
- For filling:
- 1 tbsp butter, softened
- 2 tbsp Swerve
- 3 tbsp creamy peanut butter

Directions:

1. Preheat your waffle maker.
2. In a bowl, whisk together egg, espresso powder, chocolate chips, Swerve, and cocoa powder.
3. Add mozzarella cheese and stir well.
4. Spray waffle maker with cooking spray.
5. Pour 1/2 of the batter in the hot waffle maker and cook for 3-4 minutes or until golden brown. Repeat with the remaining batter.
6. For filling: In a small bowl, stir together butter, Swerve, and peanut butter until smooth.
7. Once chaffles is cool, then spread filling mixture between two chaffle and place in the fridge for 10 minutes.
8. Cut chaffle sandwich in half and serve.

110.Chicken Chaffle Sandwich

Preparation Time: 5 minutes
Cooking Time: 15 minutes
Servings: 2

Ingredients:

- 1 chicken breast fillet, sliced into strips

- Salt and pepper to taste
- 1 teaspoon dried rosemary
- 1 tablespoon olive oil
- 4 basic chaffles
- 2 tablespoons butter, melted
- 2 tablespoons Parmesan cheese, grated

Directions:

1. Season the chicken strips with salt, pepper and rosemary.
2. Add olive oil to a pan over medium low heat.
3. Cook the chicken until brown on both sides.
4. Spread butter on top of each chaffle.
5. Sprinkle cheese on top.
6. Place the chicken on top and top with another chaffle.

111. LT Chaffle Sandwich

Preparation Time: 10 minutes
Cooking Time: 15 minutes
Servings: 2

Ingredients:

- Cooking spray
- 4 slices bacon
- 1 tablespoon mayonnaise
- 4 basic chaffles
- 2 lettuce leaves
- 2 tomato slices

Directions:

1. Coat your pan with foil and place it over medium heat.
2. Cook the bacon until golden and crispy.
3. Spread mayo on top of the chaffle.

4. Top with the lettuce, bacon and tomato.
5. Top with another chaffle.

112. Breakfast Chaffle Sandwich

Preparation Time: 10 minutes
Cooking Time: 10 minutes
Serving: 1

Ingredients:

- 2 basics cooked chaffles
- Cooking spray
- 2 slices bacon
- 1 egg

Directions:

1. Spray your pan with oil.
2. Place it over medium heat.
3. Cook the bacon until golden and crispy.
4. Put the bacon on top of one chaffle.
5. In the same pan, cook the egg without mixing until the yolk is set.
6. Add the egg on top of the bacon.
7. Top with another chaffle.

113. Sausage & Egg Chaffle Sandwich

Preparation Time: 5 minutes
Cooking Time: 10 minutes
Serving: 1

Ingredients:

- 2 basics cooked chaffles
- 1 tablespoon olive oil
- 1 sausage, sliced into rounds
- 1 egg

Directions:

1. Pour olive oil into your pan over

medium heat.

2. Put it over medium heat.

3. Add the sausage and cook until brown on both sides.

4. Put the sausage rounds on top of one chaffle.

5. Cook the egg in the same pan without mixing.

6. Place on top of the sausage rounds.

7. Top with another chaffle.

114.Bacon, Egg & Avocado Chaffle Sandwich

Preparation Time: 5 minutes
Cooking Time: 10 minutes
Servings: 2

Ingredients:

- Cooking spray
- 4 slices bacon
- 2 eggs
- ½ avocado, mashed
- 4 basic chaffles
- 2 leaves lettuce

Directions:

1. Coat your skillet with cooking spray.

2. Cook the bacon until golden and crisp.

3. Transfer into a paper towel lined plate.

4. Crack the eggs into the same pan and cook until firm.

5. Flip and cook until the yolk is set.

6. Spread the avocado on the chaffle.

7. Top with lettuce, egg and bacon.

8. Top with another chaffle.

115.Open-Faced Ham & Green Bell

Pepper Chaffle Sandwich

Preparation Time: 10 minutes
Cooking Time: 10 minutes
Servings: 2

Ingredients:

- 2 slices ham
- Cooking spray
- 1 green bell pepper, sliced into strips
- 2 slices cheese
- 1 tablespoon black olives, pitted and sliced
- 2 basic chaffles

Directions:

1. Cook the ham in a pan coated with oil over medium heat.

2. Next, cook the bell pepper.

3. Assemble the open-faced sandwich by topping each chaffle with ham and cheese, bell pepper and olives.

4. Toast in the oven until the cheese has melted a little.

116.Sausage & Pepperoni Chaffle Sandwich

Preparation Time: 10 minutes
Cooking Time: 10 minutes
Servings: 4

Ingredients:

- Cooking spray
- 2 cervelat sausage, sliced into rounds
- pieces pepperoni
- 6 mushroom slices
- 4 teaspoons mayonnaise
- 4 big white onion rings
- 4 basic chaffles

Directions:

1. Spray your skillet with oil.

2. Place over medium heat.

3. Cook the sausage until brown on both sides.

4. Transfer on a plate.

5. Cook the pepperoni and mushrooms for 2 minutes.

6. Spread mayo on top of the chaffle.

7. Top with the sausage, pepperoni, mushrooms and onion rings.

8. Top with another chaffle.

117.Keto Ice Cream Sandwich Chaffle

Preparation Time: 5 minutes
Cooking Time: 5 minutes
Servings: 2

Ingredients

- 2 Tbs cocoa
- 2 Tbs Monkfruit Confectioner's
- 1 egg
- 1/4 teaspoon baking powder
- 1 Tbs Heavy Whipped Cream
- Add selected keto ice cream

Directions:

1. Whip the egg in a small bowl.

2. Add the rest of the ingredients and mix well until smooth and creamy.

3. Pour half of the batter into a mini waffle maker and cook until fully cooked for 2 1/2 to 3 minutes.

4. Allow the ice cream to cool completely before ice cream is placed in the center.

5. Freeze all the way to solid.

6. Serve and bear the weather!

Low Carb Mini Pizza Chaffle

Preparation time: 5 minutes
Cooking time: 5 minutes
Servings: 2

Ingredients:

- 1 egg
- 1/2 cup mozzarella cheese shredded
- 1/4 teaspoon of garlic powder
- 1/2 tsp Italian seasoning
- Salt and pepper
- Toppings
- (Tomato sauce, cheese, pepperoni, etc)

Directions:

1. Put all ingredients in a bowl. Mix well.

2. Preheat the waffle maker. When it's hot, spray olive oil and put half of the dough in a mini waffle maker or put all dough in a large waffle maker. Cook each chaffle for 2-4 minutes.

3. Add the toppings and bake or fry the mini pizza until the cheese topping has melted. Serve and enjoy!

118.Pepperoni Pizza Chaffle

Preparation time: 5 minutes
Cooking time: 10 minutes
Servings: 2

Ingredients:

- For chaffle
- 1/2 cup of mozzarella
- 1 grade A large egg
- 1 tablespoon almond flour
- 1 tsp oregano
- 1 tsp garlic powder

- 1 teaspoon baking powder
- 1 teaspoon red pepper flakes
- 6 pepperonis
- For sauce
- 1/2 tbsp tomato paste
- 1 Olive oil light rain (to make the paste a little thinner)
- A pinch of oregano

Directions:

1. Mix egg, almond meal, garlic powder, oregano, red pepper flakes, and baking powder together in a bowl.

2. Add the mozzarella cheese and coat with the mixture evenly.

3. Spray your waffle maker with oil (if necessary) and heat it up to its maximum setting.

4. Cook the waffle; check it every 5 minutes until it becomes golden and crunchy.

5. While it's cooking the chaffle, To make the sauce, mix the tomato paste, olive oil and oregano. If your sauce is too thick, it will be helped by a teaspoon of water.

6. Cut the chaffle and apply the sauce to the tomato.

7. Sprinkle on top with mozarella cheese and top with pepperonis.

8. Microwave to melt the cheese and cook the pepperonis for 30 seconds

9. Get out and enjoy yourself!

10. NOTES The information on your nutrition may vary depending on the cheese you are using. Depending on your own ingredients, measure the macros.

11. It can overflow the waffle maker, rendering it a sloppy operation. I suggest you put down a silpat mat to make it easy to clean.

12. This is going to make four mini chaffles, or two big chaffles. You can also use this as an extra big chaffle in a belguim waffle maker. Macros are a large chaffle for one.

13. Yes, you can replace almond flour with coconut flour. You can get a different texture and a drier waffle.

14. These are best enjoyed from the waffle iron, but without the toppings you can freeze just the chaffle.

119.Keto Chaffle Pizza

Preparation time: 5 minutes
Cooking time: 5 minutes
Servings: 2

Ingredients

- 1 egg
- 1/2 cup mozzarella cheese shredded
- Just a pinch of Italian seasoning
- Pizza sauce with about 1 tablespoon of sugar
- Top with shredded cheese pepperoni (or favorite topping)

Directions:

1. Preheat the waffle maker from Dash.

2. Whip the egg and seasoning together in a small bowl.

3. Mix together the shredded cheese.

4. Fill the preheated waffle maker with a tsp of shredded cheese and let it cook for about 30 seconds. This is going to help create a crisper crust.

5. Add half of the mixture to the waffle maker and cook until golden brown and mildly crispy for about 4 minutes!

6. Cut the waffle to make the second chaffle and add the remaining mixture

to the waffle maker.

01. Finish with a pasta sauce teaspoon, shredded cheese and pepperoni. For about 20 seconds, microwave it on top and voila! Instant PIZZA Chaffle!

120.Chaffle Bagel

Preparation time: 5 minutes
Cooking time: 5 minutes
We all love bagels, the round/doughnut shaped type of bread. You can make your own Chaffle based bagel with this recipe.

Ingredients

- 1 large egg
- 1 tsp of coconut flour
- 1 tsp of Bagel seasoning
- 1/2 cup of shredded mozzarella
- 2 tsp of cream cheese for serving.

Directions

1. First step is to pre-heat the mini waffle iron.

2. Then you whisk the egg in a bowl with the bagel seasoning, coconut flour then stir in the cheese.

3. Spread half of the egg you have mixed with the other ingredients into the waffle iron and allow it to cook for about 3 minutes. Then you remove the waffle and repeat the steps with the remaining egg mixture. Next step is to spread each bagel waffle with cream cheese. You can also sprinkle additional bagel seasoning.

121.Bruleed French Toast Chaffle Monte Cristo

Preparation time: 5 minutes
Cooking time: 10 minutes
Servings: 1

Ingredients:

- For the chaffles:
- 1 egg
- 1/8 tsp baking powder
- 1/4 tsp cinnamon
- 1/2 tsp monkfruit
- 1 tbsp cream cheese
- 2 tsp brown sugar substitute
- For the filling:
- 2 oz deli ham
- 2 oz deli turkey
- 1 slice provolone cheese
- 1/2 tsp sugar-free jelly

Directions:

1. Preheat the waffle maker.

2. Place all the chaffle ingredients, except the sugar substitute, inside a blender. Make sure to place the cream cheese closest to the blades. Blend the ingredients until you achieve a smooth consistency.

3. Sprinkle the waffle maker with 1/2 tsp of brown sugar substitute.

4. Onto the waffle maker, pour 1/2 of the batter. Sprinkle another 1/2 teaspoon of the brown sugar substitute.

5. Close the lid and allow the batter to cook for 3-5 minutes.

6. Remove the chaffle. Repeat the steps until you used up all the batter.

7. Prepare the chaffle by spreading jelly on one surface of the chaffle.

8. Following this order, place the ham, turkey, and cheese in a small, microwaveable bowl. Place inside the microwave. Heat until the cheese is melted.

9. Invert the bowl onto the chaffle so

that the contents transfer onto the chaffle. The cheese should be under the ham and turkey, directly sitting on top of the chaffle.

01. Top with the other chaffle and flip it over before serving.

122.Lemon Chaffle Dome Cake

Preparation time: 30 minutes
Cooking time: 30 minutes
Servings: 4

Ingredients:

- For the chaffles:
- 2 eggs
- 2 oz cream cheese, softened
- 1 tbsp coconut flour
- 2 tsp heavy cream
- 2 tsp lemon juice
- 1/2 tsp vanilla extract
- 1/4 tsp stevia powder
- 1/4 tsp baking soda
- For the lemon frosting:
- 8 oz cream cheese, softened
- 2 oz unsalted butter, softened
- 1 tbsp stevia powder
- 1 tbsp lemon zest
- 1 tsp lemon juice
- 1/2 tsp vanilla extract

Directions:

1. Preheat the mini waffle maker.
2. Combine all the chaffle ingredients using a blender.
3. Onto the preheated waffle maker, pour 1/4 of the batter.
4. Close the lid. Let the batter cook for 4-5 minutes. Remove the

cooked chaffle using a pair of silicone tongs.

5. Repeat the steps to use up the remaining batter.
6. Let the chaffles cool completely.
7. Make the lemon frosting by combining the ingredients in a bowl.
8. Assemble by cutting two of the chaffles in half.
9. Use cling wrap to line a small bowl.
10. Place a whole chaffle in the bowl, carefully molding it to the shape of the bowl.
11. Line each side with the four chaffle halves.
12. Add half the amount of lemon frosting.
13. Cover the frosting with the last whole chaffle.
14. Cover the bowl with cling wrap. Put in the fridge for 30 minutes. You don't need to chill the remaining lemon frosting.
15. Invert the chaffle dome onto a plate.
16. Spread the remaining lemon frosting over it. Add decorations if desired.
17. Chill the cake for another 30 minutes. Serve.

123.Keema Curry Chaffle

Preparation time: 10 minutes
Cooking time: 5 minutes
Servings: 4

Ingredients:

- For the chaffles:
- 2 eggs

- 3 oz mozzarella cheese, shredded
- 3 tbsp almond flour
- 1/2 tsp baking powder
- 1/4 tsp garlic powder
- For the keema curry:
- oz ground beef
- 1 tbsp avocado oil
- 1/4 tsp salt
- 1/2 tsp garlic powder
- 1/4 tsp ginger powder
- 1/2 cup tomato puree
- 2 tbsp curry powder
- 2 tbsp Worcestershire sauce
- For the topping:
- 4 tsp parmesan cheese, finely grated

Directions:

1. Start by making the curry, over medium heat, heat avocado oil in a frying pan.
2. Add in the ground meat and cook until it turns brown.
3. Add the ginger powder, garlic powder, and salt. Stir well.
4. Stir in the Worcestershire sauce and the tomato puree.
5. Finally, add the curry powder and stir it in.
6. Allow to simmer for about 6-10 minutes over low heat.
7. Preheat the mini waffle maker.
8. Combine all chaffle ingredients, except cheese, in a small mixing bowl.
9. Sprinkle some cheese onto the heated waffle maker and let it melt.
10. When the cheese melts, immediately pour 1/4 of the batter on top of it.

Spread 2 tsp of keema curry then sprinkle some more cheese.

11. Close the lid. Cook for 4 minutes.
12. Remove the cooked chaffle and repeat the steps until you've used up all the batter.
13. Once all chaffles are cooked, use the remaining keema curry on top.
14. Top all the chaffles with parmesan cheese.

124. Garlic Bread Chaffle

Preparation Time: 5 min
Cooking Time: 4 min
Servings: 2

Ingredients:

- 1 clove Garlic, grated
- 1/2 tsp Italian seasoning
- 1/4 tsp Baking powder
- 1 large Egg
- 1/3 cup Parmesan cheese, grated
- 1/2 cup shredded Mozzarella cheese

Directions:

1. Preheat mini waffle maker for about 5 minutes until hot.
2. Add cheese and egg to a small bowl and combine thoroughly. Stir in the remaining ingredients (except toppings).
3. Pour ½ of the batter into the waffle maker and spread well.
4. Cook until a bit browned and crispy, about 4 minutes.
5. Gently remove from waffle maker and set aside for 2 minutes so it cools down and become crispy
6. Repeat with remaining batter.
7. Top with extra melted cheese

Nutrition:

182 calories
2g net carbs
11g fat
16g protein

125.Cinnamon 'Churro' Chaffle

Preparation Time: 5 min
Cooking Time: 4 min
Servings: 2

Ingredients:

- 3/4 tsp Cinnamon (for topping)
- 2 tbsp almond flour
- 1 large Egg
- 1/2 tbsp Butter, melted
- 1/2 tsp Cinnamon
- 1 tbsp Butter, melted (for topping)
- 3/4 cup Mozzarella cheese (shredded)
- 2 tbsp Erythritol
- 1/4 tsp Baking powder (optional)
- 1/2 tsp Vanilla extract
- 1 tsp psyllium husk powder

Directions:

1. Preheat mini waffle maker for about 5 minutes until hot.

2. Add cheese and egg to a small bowl and combine thoroughly. Stir in the remaining ingredients (except toppings, if any).

3. Pour ½ of the batter into the waffle maker; spread evenly

4. Cook until a bit browned and crispy, about 4 minutes.

5. Gently remove from waffle maker and set aside for 2 minutes so it cools down to become crispy.

6. Repeat with remaining batter.

7. Brush with melted butter and sprinkle with cinnamon "sugar" topping

8. Cut into churro sticks if so desired

Nutrition:

179 calories
2g net carbs
14g fat
10g protein

126.Pumpkin Pie Chaffle

Preparation Time: 5 min
Cooking Time: 4 min
Servings: 2

Ingredients:

- 1/2 cup Mozzarella cheese (shredded)
- 1 large Egg
- 2 1/2 tbsp Erythritol
- 1/2 oz Cream cheese
- 3 tsp Coconut flour
- 2 tbsp Pumpkin puree
- 1/4 tsp Baking powder (optional)
- 1/2 tbsp Pumpkin pie spice
- 1/2 tsp Vanilla extract (optional)
- 2 tbsp Heavy whipping cream (topping)
- Dash of cinnamon (topping)

Directions:

1. Preheat mini waffle maker until hot

2. Whisk egg in a bowl, add cheese, then mix well

3. Stir in the remaining ingredients (except toppings, if any).

4. Pour half of the batter onto the waffle maker, spread evenly

5. Cook until a bit browned and crispy, about 4 minutes.

6. Gently remove from waffle maker and let it cool

7. Repeat with remaining batter.

8. Top with whipped cream and cinnamon

Nutrition:

117 calories
3g net carbs
7g fat
7g protein

127.Spicy Flavored Chaffle

Preparation Time: 5 min
Cooking Time: 4 min
Servings: 2

Ingredients:

- 1 cup Cheddar cheese (shredded)
- 1 large Egg
- 1 oz Cream cheese
- 2 tbsp Bacon bits
- 2 Jalapenos, sliced
- 1/4 tsp Baking powder (optional)

Directions:

1. Preheat mini waffle maker until hot

2. Whisk egg in a bowl, add cheese, then mix well

3. Stir in the remaining ingredients (except toppings, if any).

4. Scoop 1/2 of the batter onto the waffle maker, spread across evenly

5. Cook 3-4 minutes, until done as desired (or crispy).

6. Gently remove from waffle maker and let it cool

7. Repeat with remaining batter.

8. Top with melted cheese, jalapeno slices, and bacon bits

Nutrition:

231 calories
2g net carbs
18g fat
13g protein

128.Keto Seasoned Chaffle

Preparation Time: 5 min
Cooking Time: 4 min
Servings: 2

Ingredients:

- 1 large egg
- 1/2 c. shredded cheese
- Pinch of salt
- Seasoning to taste

Directions:

1. Preheat mini waffle maker until hot

2. Whisk egg in a bowl, add cheese, then mix well

3. Stir in the remaining ingredients (except toppings, if any).

4. Scoop ½ of the batter onto the waffle maker, spread across evenly

5. Cook until a bit browned and crispy, about 4 minutes.

6. Gently remove from waffle maker and let it cool

7. Repeat with remaining batter.

8. Enjoy!

Nutrition:

241 calories
2g net carbs
19g fat
12g protein

129.Keto Chaffle With Cream

Preparation Time: 5 min
Cooking Time: 4 min

Servings: 2

Ingredients:

- 1 large egg
- 1/2 cup shredded mozzarella
- 1 tbsp of almond flour
- 1 tsp vanilla
- 1 shake of cinnamon
- 1/2 tsp baking powder
- 1/2 tbsp whipped cream

Directions:

1. Preheat mini waffle maker until hot
2. Whisk egg in a bowl, add cheese, then mix well
3. Stir in the remaining ingredients (except toppings, if any).
4. Scoop ½ of the batter on the waffle maker, spread across evenly
5. Cook until a bit browned and crispy, about 4 minutes.
6. Cook 3-4 minutes, until done as desired (or crispy).
7. Gently remove from waffle maker and let it cool
8. Repeat with remaining batter.
9. Top with whipped cream and cinnamon

Nutrition:

271 calories
2g net carbs
27g fat
13g protein

130.Sweet & Spicy Chaffle

Preparation Time: 5 min
Cooking Time: 4 min
Servings: 2

Ingredients:

- 1 large egg
- 1/2 cup mozzarella cheese
- 2 tbsp Stevia, liquid
- 1/2 tsp salt
- 1/2 tsp smoked paprika
- Pinch of cayenne pepper

Directions:

1. Preheat mini waffle maker until hot
2. Whisk egg in a bowl, add cheese, then mix well
3. Stir in the remaining ingredients (except toppings, if any).
4. Scoop 1/2 of the batter onto the waffle maker, spread across evenly
5. Cook 3-4 minutes, until done as desired (or crispy).
6. Gently remove from waffle maker and let it cool
7. Repeat with remaining batter.
8. Top with whipped cream and cinnamon

Nutrition:

252 calories
3g net carbs
21g fat
12g protein

131.Savory Herb Chaffle

Preparation Time: 5 min
Cooking Time: 4 min
Servings: 2

Ingredients:

- 1 large egg
- 1/4 cup shredded mozzarella
- 1/4 cup shredded parmesan
- 1/2 tbsp butter, melted

- 1 tsp herb blend seasoning
- 1/2 tsp salt

Directions:

1. Preheat mini waffle maker until hot
2. Whisk egg in a bowl, add cheese, then mix well
3. Stir in the remaining ingredients (except toppings, if any).
4. Scoop 1/2 of the batter onto the waffle maker, spread across evenly
5. Cook until a bit browned and crispy, about 4 minutes.
6. Cook 3-4 minutes, until done as desired (or crispy).
7. Gently remove from waffle maker and let it cool
8. Repeat with remaining batter.
9. Serve and Enjoy!

Nutrition:

294 calories
2g net carbs
24g fat
12g protein

132Hot Brown Sandwich Chaffle

Preparation time: 15 minutes
Cooking time: 5 minutes
Servings: 2

Ingredients:

- For the chaffles:
- 1 egg, beaten
- 1/4 cup cheddar cheese, shredded and divided
- For the sandwich:
- 2 slices fresh tomato
- 1/2 lb roasted turkey breast
- 1/2 tsp parmesan cheese, grated

- 2 bacon, cooked
- For the sauce:
- 2 oz cream cheese, cubed
- 1/3 cup heavy cream
- 1/4 cup swiss cheese, shredded
- 1/4 tsp ground nutmeg
- White pepper

Directions:

1. Preheat the waffle maker.
2. Start by making the chaffle, once heated up, sprinkle 1 tbsp cheddar cheese onto the iron.
3. After 30 seconds, top the cheese with beaten egg.
4. Once the egg starts to cook, top the mixture with another layer of cheese.
5. Close the waffle maker lid and allow to cook for 3-5 minutes until the chaffle is crispy and golden brown.
6. Take out the cooked chaffle and repeat the steps until you've used up all the batter.
7. Make the sauce by combining heavy cream and cream cheese in a small saucepan.
8. Place saucepan over medium heat and whisk until the cheese completely dissolves.
9. Add in Swiss cheese and parmesan, then continue whisking to melt the cheese.
10. Add in the white pepper and nutmeg.
11. Continue whisking until you achieve a smooth consistency.
12. Remove the sauce pan from heat.
13. Prepare the sandwich by setting

the oven for broiling.

14. Cover a cookie sheet with aluminum foil.

15. Lightly grease the foil with butter, and place two chaffles on it.

16. Top the chaffles with 4 oz of turkey and a slice of tomato each. Add some sauce and grated parmesan on top.

17. Broil the chaffle sandwiches for 2-3 minutes until you see the sauce bubble and brown spots appear on top.

18. Remove from the oven. Put them on a heatproof plate.

19. Arrange bacon slices in a crisscross manner on top of the sandwich before serving.

01. Nutrition: Calories: 572 Carbohydrates: 3g Fat: 41g Protein: 41g

133.Strawberry Cream Sandwich Chaffles

Preparation time: 10 minutes
Cooking time: 6 minutes
Servings: 2

Ingredients

- Chaffles
- 1 large organic egg, beaten
- ½ cup mozzarella cheese, shredded finely
- Filling
- 4 teaspoons heavy cream
- 2 tablespoons powdered erythritol
- 1 teaspoon fresh lemon juice
- Pinch of fresh lemon zest, grated
- 2 fresh strawberries, hulled and sliced

Directions:

1. Preheat a mini waffle iron and then grease it.

2. For chaffles: in a small bowl, add the egg and mozzarella cheese and stir to combine.

3. Place half of the mixture into preheated waffle iron and cook for about 2–3 minutes.

4. Repeat with the remaining mixture.

5. Meanwhile, for filling: in a bowl, Place all the ingredients except the strawberry slices and with a hand mixer, beat until well combined.

6. Serve each chaffle with cream mixture and strawberry slices.

134.Strawberry Cream Cheese Sandwich Chaffles

Preparation time: 15 minutes
Cooking time: 10 minutes
Servings: 2

Ingredients

- Chaffles
- 1 organic egg, beaten
- 1 teaspoon organic vanilla extract
- 1 tablespoon almond flour
- 1 teaspoon organic baking powder
- Pinch of ground cinnamon
- 1 cup mozzarella cheese, shredded
- Filling
- 2 tablespoons cream cheese, softened
- 2 tablespoons erythritol
- ¼ teaspoon organic vanilla extract
- 2 fresh strawberries, hulled and chopped

Directions:

1. Preheat a mini waffle iron and then grease it.

2. For chaffles: in a bowl, add the egg and vanilla extract and mix well.

3. Add the flour, baking powder, and cinnamon, and mix until well combined.

4. Add the mozzarella cheese and stir to combine.

5. Place half of the mixture into preheated waffle iron and cook for about 4–5 minutes.

6. Repeat with the remaining mixture.

7. Meanwhile, for filling: in a bowl, Place all the ingredients except the strawberry pieces and with a hand mixer, beat until well combined.

8. Serve each chaffle with cream cheese mixture and strawberry pieces.

135.Blueberry Peanut Butter Sandwich Chaffles

Preparation time: 10 minutes
Cooking time: 10 minutes
Servings: 2

Ingredients

- 1 organic egg, beaten
- ½ cup cheddar cheese, shredded
- Filling
- 2 tablespoons erythritol
- 1 tablespoon butter, softened
- 1 tablespoon natural peanut butter
- 2 tablespoons cream cheese, softened
- ¼ teaspoon organic vanilla extract
- 2 teaspoons fresh blueberries

Directions:

1. Preheat a mini waffle iron and then grease it.

2. For chaffles: in a small bowl, add the egg and Cheddar cheese and stir to combine.

3. Place half of the mixture into preheated waffle iron and cook for about 3–5 minutes.

4. Repeat with the remaining mixture.

5. Meanwhile, for filling: In a medium bowl, put all ingredients and mix until well combined.

6. Serve each chaffle with peanut butter mixture.

136.French Dip Keto Chaffle Sandwich

Preparation Time: 5 mins
Cooking Time: 12 mins
Servings: 2

Ingredients:

- 1 egg white
- 1/4 cup mozzarella cheese, shredded (packed)
- 1/4 cup sharp cheddar cheese, shredded (packed)
- 3/4 tsp water
- 1 tsp coconut flour
- 1/4 tsp baking powder
- Pinch of salt

Directions:

1. Preheat oven to 425 degrees. Plug the Dash Mini Waffle Maker in the wall and grease lightly once it is hot.

2. Combine all of the ingredients in a bowl and stir to combine.

3. Spoon out 1/2 of the batter on the waffle maker and close lid. Set a timer for 4 minutes and do not lift the lid until the cooking time is complete. Lifting beforehand can cause the Chaffle keto sandwich recipe to

separate and stick to the waffle iron. You have to let it cook the entire 4 minutes before lifting the lid.

4. Remove the chaffle from the waffle iron and set aside. Repeat the same steps above with the rest of the chaffle batter.

5. Cover a cookie sheet with parchment paper and place chaffles a few inches apart.

6. Add 1/4 to 1/3 cup of the slow cooker keto roast beef from the following recipe. Make sure to drain the excess broth/gravy before adding to the top of the chaffle.

7. Add a slice of deli cheese or shredded cheese on top. Swiss and provolone are both great options.

8. Place on the top rack of the oven for 5 minutes so that the cheese can melt. If you'd like the cheese to bubble and begin to brown, turn oven to broil for 1 min. (The swiss cheese may not brown)

9. Enjoy open-faced with a small bowl of beef broth for dipping.

DESSERT CHAFFLES

137. Chocolatey Chaffle

Preparation Time: 5 min
Cooking Time: 4 min
Servings: 2

Ingredients:

- 1 large egg
- 1 oz. cream cheese, softened
- 1 tbsp ChocZero Chocolate Syrup
- 1/2 tsp vanilla
- 1 tbsp Stevia sweetener
- 1/2 tbsp cacao powder
- 1/4 tsp baking powder

Directions:

2. Preheat mini waffle maker until hot
3. Whisk egg in a bowl, add cheese, then mix well
4. Stir in the remaining ingredients (except toppings, if any).
5. Scoop 1/2 of the batter onto the waffle maker, spread across evenly
6. Cook until a bit browned and crispy, about 4 minutes.
7. Gently remove from waffle maker and let it cool
8. Repeat with remaining batter.
9. Serve and Enjoy!

Nutrition:

241 calories
2g net carbs
19g fat
13g protein

138. Keto Chocolate Chip Chaffle

Preparation Time: 5 min
Cooking Time: 8 min
Servings: 1

Ingredients

- 1 egg
- 1/4 tsp baking powder
- Pinch of salt
- 1 tbsp heavy whipping cream (topping)
- 1/2 tsp coconut flour
- 1 tbsp Chocolate Chips

Directions:

1. Preheat mini waffle maker until hot
2. Whisk egg in a bowl, add cheese, then mix well
3. Stir in the remaining ingredients (except toppings, if any).
4. Grease preheated waffle maker with. This will help to create a more crisp crust.
5. Scoop 1/2 of the batter onto the waffle maker, spread across evenly.
6. Sprinkle chocolate chips on top
7. Cook until a bit browned and crispy, about 4 minutes.
8. Gently remove from waffle maker and let it cool
9. Repeat with remaining batter.
10. Top with whipping cream
11. Serve and Enjoy!

Nutrition:

146 calories
3g net carbs
10g fat

6g protein

139. Chocolate Chip Cannoli Chaffles

Preparation time: 15 minutes
Cooking time: 5 minutes
Servings: 4

Ingredients:

- For the chocolate chip chaffle:
- 1 tbsp butter, melted
- 1 tbsp monkfruit
- 1 egg yolk
- 1/8 tsp vanilla extract
- 3 tbsp almond flour
- 1/8 tsp baking powder
- 1 tbsp chocolate chips, sugar-free
- For the cannoli topping:
- 2 oz cream cheese
- 2 tbsp low-carb confectioners sweetener
- 6 tbsp ricotta cheese, full fat
- 1/4 tsp vanilla extract
- 5 drops lemon extract

Directions:

1. Preheat the mini waffle maker.
2. Mix all the ingredients for the chocolate chip chaffle in a mixing bowl. Combine well to make a batter.
3. Place half the batter on the waffle maker. Allow to cook for 3-4 minutes.
4. While waiting for the chaffles to cook, start making your cannoli topping by combining all ingredients until the consistency is creamy and smooth.
5. Place the cannoli topping on the cooked chaffles before serving.

Nutrition: Calories: 187 Carbohydrates: 7g

Fat: 13g Protein: 7g

140. Oreo Chaffle

Preparation time: 10 minutes
Cooking time: 20 minutes
Servings: 2

Ingredients:

- 2 teaspoons coconut flour
- 3 tablespoons cocoa, unsweetened
- 1 teaspoon baking powder
- 4 tablespoons swerve sweetener
- 1 teaspoon vanilla extract, unsweetened
- 2 tablespoons heavy cream
- 2 eggs, at room temperature
- 2 tablespoons whipped cream

Directions:

1. Take a non-stick waffle iron, plug it in, select the medium or medium-high heat setting and let it preheat until ready to use; it could also be indicated with an indicator light changing its color.
2. Meanwhile, prepare the batter and for this, take a large bowl, add flour in it along with other ingredients and mix with an electric mixer until smooth.
3. Use a ladle to pour one-fourth of the prepared batter into the heated waffle iron in a spiral direction, starting from the edges, then shut the lid and cook for 5 minutes or more until solid and nicely browned; the cooked waffle will look like a cake.
4. When done, transfer chaffles to a plate with a silicone spatula and repeat with the remaining batter.
5. When done, prepare the oreo sandwiches, and for this, spread 1 tablespoon of whipped cream on one

side of two chaffles and then cover with the remaining chaffles.

6. Serve immediately.

141. Brownie Batter Chaffle

Preparation time: 10 minutes
Cooking time: 25 minutes
Servings: 16

Ingredients:

- 1/2 cup / 50 grams almond flour
- ½ cup / 75 grams chopped chocolate, unsweetened
- 1 teaspoon baking powder
- 1/4 teaspoon salt
- 1/4 cup / 40 grams cocoa powder, unsweetened
- 1/4 teaspoon liquid stevia
- 1/2 cup / 100 grams Swerve Sweetener
- 1/2 teaspoon vanilla extract, unsweetened
- 12 tablespoons coconut butter
- 5 eggs, at room temperature

Directions:

1. Take a non-stick waffle iron, plug it in, select the medium or medium-high heat setting and let it preheat until ready to use; it could also be indicated with an indicator light changing its color.

2. Meanwhile, prepare the batter and for this, take a saucepan, place it over medium heat, add cocoa powder, chocolate, and butter and cook for 3 to 4 minutes until the butter has melted, whisking frequently.

3. Then add sweetener, stevia, and vanilla into the pan, stir until combined, remove the pan from heat

and let it stand for 5 minutes.

4. Take a medium bowl, add flour in it and then stir in baking powder and salt until mixed.

5. After 5 minutes, beat eggs into the chocolate-butter mixture and stir the flour until incorporated.

6. Use a ladle to pour ¼ cup of the prepared batter into the heated waffle iron in a spiral direction, starting from the edges, then shut the lid and cook for 5 minutes or more until solid and nicely browned; the cooked waffle will look like a cake.

7. When done, transfer chaffles to a plate with a silicone spatula and repeat with the remaining batter.

8. Let chaffles stand for some time until crispy and serve straight away.

142. Fudgy Chocolate Chaffles

Preparation Time: 5 mins
Cooking Time: 8 mins
Servings: 2

Ingredients:

- 1 egg
- 2 tbsp mozzarella cheese, shredded
- 2 tbsp cocoa
- 2 tbsp Lakanto monk fruit powdered
- 1 tsp coconut flour
- 1 tsp heavy whipping cream
- 1/4 tsp baking powder
- 1/4 tsp vanilla extract
- pinch of salt

Directions:

1. Turn on waffle or chaffle maker. I use the Dash Mini Waffle Maker. Grease lightly or use a cooking spray.

2. In a small bowl, combine all ingredients.

3. Cover the dash mini waffle maker with 1/2 of the batter. Close the mini waffle maker and cook for 4 minutes. Remove the chaffle from the waffle maker carefully as it is very hot.

4. Repeat the steps above.

5. Serve with sugar-free strawberry ice cream or sugar-free whipped topping.

143.Keto Cornbread Chaffle

Preparation time: 10 minutes
Cooking time: 5 minutes

Ingredients:

- 1 egg
- 1/2 cup cheddar cheese shredded (or mozzarella)
- 5 slices jalapeno optional - picked or fresh
- 1 tsp Frank's Red hot sauce
- 1/4 tsp corn extract
- pinch salt

Directions:

1. Preheat the mini waffle maker

2. In a small bowl, whip the egg.

3. Add the remaining ingredients and mix it until it's well incorporated.

4. Add a teaspoon of shredded cheese to the waffle maker for 30 seconds before adding the mixture. This will create a nice and crisp crust that is absolutely fantastic!

5. Add half the mixture to the preheated waffle maker.

6. Cook it for a minimum of 3 to 4 minutes. The longer you cook it, the crispier it gets.

7. Serve warm and enjoy!

144.Crispy Bagel Chaffle Chips

Preparation time: 10 minutes
Cooking time: 5 minutes
Serving: 1

Ingredients:

- 3 Tbs Parmesan cheese shredded
- 1 tsp Everything Bagel Seasoning

Directions:

1. Preheat the mini waffle maker.

2. Place the Parmesan cheese on the griddle and allow it to bubble. About 3 minutes. Be sure to leave it long enough, or else it won't turn crispy when it cools. Important step!

3. Sprinkle the melted cheese with about 1 teaspoon of Everything Bagel Seasoning. Leave the waffle iron open when it cooks!

4. Unplug the mini waffle maker and allow it to cool for a few minutes. This will allow the cheese to cool enough to bind together and get crispy.

5. After about 2 minutes of it cooling off, it will still be warm.

6. Use a mini spatula to peel the warm (but not hot cheese from the mini waffle iron.

7. Allow it to cool completely for crispy chips! These chips pack a powerful crunch, which is something I tend to miss on Keto!

145.Lime Pie Chaffle Recipe

Preparation time: 10 minutes
Cooking time: 5 minutes
Serving: 2

Ingredients:

- Key Lime Pie Chaffle Recipe ingredients:
- 1 egg
- 1/4 cup Almond flour
- 2 tsp cream cheese room temp
- 1 tsp powdered sweetener swerve or monk fruit
- 1/2 tsp lime extract or 1 tsp fresh squeezed lime juice
- 1/2 tsp baking powder
- 1/2 tsp lime zest
- Pinch of salt to bring out the flavors
- Cream Cheese Lime Frosting Ingredients:
- 4 oz cream cheese softened
- 4 tbs butter
- 2 tsp powdered sweetener swerve or monk fruit
- 1 tsp lime extract
- 1/2 tsp lime zest

Directions:

1. Preheat the mini waffle iron.
2. In a blender, add all the chaffle ingredients and blend on high until the mixture is smooth and creamy.
3. Cook each chaffle about 3 to 4 minutes until it's golden brown.
4. While the chaffles are cooking, make the frosting.
5. In a small bowl, combine all the ingredients for the frosting and mix it until it's smooth.
6. Allow the chaffles to completely cool before frosting them.
7. Optional:
8. Top with whipped cream or the cream cheese frosting. Add a small amount

of lime zest for an extra touch!

146. Keto Smores Chaffle

Preparation time: 15 minutes
Cooking time: 10 minutes
Servings: 2

Ingredients:

- 1 large Egg
- ½ c. Mozzarella cheese shredded
- ½ tsp Vanilla extract
- 2 tbs swerve brown
- ½ tbs Psyllium Husk Powder optional
- ¼ tsp Baking Powder
- Pinch of pink salt
- ¼ Lily's Original Dark Chocolate Bar
- 2 tbs Keto Marshmallow Creme Fluff Recipe

Directions:

1. Make the batch of Keto Marshmallow Creme Fluff.
2. Whisk the egg until creamy.
3. Add vanilla and Swerve Brown, mix well.
4. Mix in the shredded cheese and blend.
5. Then add Psyllium Husk Powder, baking powder, and salt.
6. Mix until well incorporated, let the batter rest 3-4 minutes.
7. Prep/plug in your waffle maker to preheat.
8. Spread ½ batter on the waffle maker and cook 3-4 minutes.
9. Remove and set on a cooling rack.
10. Cook second half of batter same, then remove to cool.
11. Once cool, assemble the chaffles with the marshmallow fluff and chocolate:

12. Using 2 tbs marshmallow and ¼ bar of Lily's Chocolate.

13. Eat as is, or toast for a melty and gooey Smore sandwich!

147. Keto Vanilla Twinkie Copycat Chaffle Recipe

Preparation time: 10 minutes
Cooking time: 4 minutes
Servings: 4

Ingredients:

- 2 tablespoons butter melted (cooled)

- 2 ounces cream cheese softened

- 2 large eggs room temp

- 1 teaspoon vanilla extract

- 1/2 teaspoon Vanilla Cupcake Extract (optional)

- 1/4 cup Lakanto Confectioners

- Pinch of pink salt

- 1/4 cup almond flour

- 2 tablespoons coconut flour

- 1 teaspoon baking powder

Directions:

1. Preheat the Corndog Maker.

2. Melt the butter and let it cool a minute.

3. Whisk the eggs into the butter until creamy.

4. Add vanilla, extract, sweetener, salt, and then blend well.

5. Add Almond flour, coconut flour, and baking powder.

6. Blend until well incorporated.

7. Add 2 tbsp batter to each well and spread across evenly.

8. Close lid, lock, and let cook 4 minutes.

9. Remove and cool on a rack.

148. Peppermint Mocha Chaffles with Buttercream Frosting

Preparation time: 10 minutes
Cooking time: 10 minutes
Servings: 6

Ingredients:

- Chaffles:

- 1 egg

- 1 ounce cream cheese at room temperature

- 1 tablespoon melted butter or coconut oil

- 1 tablespoon unsweetened cocoa powder or raw cacao

- 2 tablespoons powdered sweeteners such as Swerve or Lakanto

- 1 tablespoon almond flour

- 2 teaspoons coconut flour

- 1/4 teaspoon baking powder powder

- 1 teaspoon instant coffee granules

- 1/4 teaspoon vanilla extract

- Pinch salt

- Filling:

- 2 tablespoons butter at room temperature

- 2-3 tablespoons powdered sweeteners such as Swerve or Lakanto

- 1/4 teaspoon vanilla extract

- 1/8 teaspoon peppermint extract

- Optional toppings: sugar-free starlight mints

Directions:

1. For the Mocha Chaffles:

2. Heat mini Dash waffle iron until thoroughly hot.

3. Beat all chaffle ingredients together in a small bowl until smooth.

4. Add a heaping 2 tablespoons of batter to waffle iron and cook until done about 4 minutes.

5. Repeat to make 3 chaffles. Let cool on wire rack.

6. For the Buttercream Frosting:

7. In a small bowl with a hand mixer, beat the butter and sweetener until smooth.

8. Add the heavy cream and vanilla extract and beat at high speed for about 4 minutes, until light and fluffy.

9. Spread frosting on each chaffle and garnish with sugar-free starlight mints, if desired.

149.Cranberry Swirl Chaffles with Orange Cream Cheese Frosting

Preparation time: 10 minutes
Cooking time: 20 minutes
Servings: 6

Ingredients:

- Cranberry sauce:
- 1/2 cup cranberries fresh or frozen
- 2 Tbsp granulated erythritol
- 1/2 cup water
- 1/2 tsp vanilla extract
- Chaffles:
- 1 egg
- 1 ounce cream cheese at room temperature
- 1 Tbsp erythritol blends such as Swerve, Pyure or Lakanto
- 1/2 tsp vanilla extract

- 1 tsp coconut flour
- 1/4 tsp baking powder
- Frosting:
- 1 ounce cream cheese at room temperature
- 1 Tbsp butter room temperature
- 1 Tbsp confectioner's sweetener such as Swerve
- 1/8 tsp orange extract OR 2 drops orange essential oil
- A few strands of grated orange zest (optional)

Directions:

1. For the cranberry swirl:

2. Combine the cranberries, water, and erythritol in a medium saucepan. Bring to a boil, then reduce heat to a gentle simmer.

3. Simmer for 10-15 minutes, until the cranberries pop and the sauce thickens.

4. Remove from heat and stir in the vanilla extract.

5. Mash the berries with the back of a spoon until a chunky sauce forms.

6. The sauce will thicken off the heat significantly.

7. For the chaffles:

8. Preheat mini Dash waffle iron until thoroughly hot.

9. In a medium bowl, whisk all chaffle ingredients together until well combined.

10. Spoon 2 tablespoons of batter into a waffle iron.

11. Add 1/2 of the cranberry sauce in little dollops over the batter of each chaffle.

12. Close and cook 3-5 minutes, until

done. Remove to a wire rack.

13. Repeat for the second chaffle.

14. For the Frosting:

15. Mix all ingredients, except orange zest, together until smooth and spread over each chaffle.

16. Orange zest (optional).

150. Zucchini Nut Bread Chaffle Recipe

Preparation time: 10 minutes
Cooking time: 15 minutes

Ingredients

- 1 cup shredded zucchini approximately 1 small zucchini
- 1 egg
- 1/2 teaspoon cinnamon
- 1 Tbsp plus 1 tsp erythritol blend such as Swerve, Pyure or Lakanto
- Dash ground nutmeg
- 2 tsp melted butter
- 1 ounce softened cream cheese
- 2 tsp coconut flour
- 1/2 tsp baking powder
- 3 tablespoons chopped walnuts or pecans
- Frosting Ingredients:
- 2 ounces cream cheese at room temperature
- 2 Tbsp butter at room temperature
- 1/4 tsp cinnamon
- 2 Tbsp caramel sugar-free syrup such as Skinny Girl, or 1 Tbsp confectioner's sweetener, such as Swerve plus 1/8 tsp caramel extract
- 1 Tbsp chopped walnuts or pecans

Directions:

1. Grate zucchini and place in a colander over a plate to drain for 15 minutes. With your hands, squeeze out as much moisture as possible.

2. Preheat mini Dash waffle iron until thoroughly hot.

3. In a medium bowl, whisk all chaffle ingredients together until well combined.

4. Spoon a heaping 2 tablespoons of batter into waffle iron, close and cook 3-5 minutes, until done.

5. Remove to a wire rack. Repeat 3 times.

6. Frosting Instructions:

7. Mix all ingredients together until smooth and spread over each chaffle.

8. Top with additional chopped nuts.

Keto Apple Fritter Chaffles

Preparation time: 30 minutes
Cooking time: 30 minutes
Servings: 5

Ingredients:

- Apple Fritter Filling Ingredients:
- 2 cups diced jicama
- 1/4 cup plus 1 tablespoon Swerve sweetener blend
- 4 tablespoons butter
- 1 teaspoon cinnamon
- 1/8 teaspoon nutmeg
- Dash ground cloves
- 1/2 teaspoon vanilla
- 20 drops Lorann Oils apple flavoring
- Chaffle Ingredients:
- 2 eggs
- 1/2 cup grated mozzarella cheese

- 1 tablespoon almond flour
- 1 teaspoon coconut flour
- 1/2 teaspoon baking powder
- Glaze Ingredients:
- 1 tablespoon butter
- 2 teaspoons heavy cream
- 3 tablespoons powdered sweetener such as Swerve Confectioners
- 1/4 teaspoon vanilla extract

Directions:

1. Keto Apple Fritter Chaffle Filling Instructions:
2. Peel the jicama and cut into small dice.
3. In a medium skillet over medium-low heat, melt the butter and add the diced jicama and sweetener.
4. Let simmer slowly for 10-20 minutes until the jicama is soft, stirring often. Do not use high heat, or the sweetener will caramelize quickly and burn. It should develop a light amber color and will thicken.
5. When the jicama is soft, remove from heat and stir in the spices and flavorings.
6. Keto Apple Fritter Chaffle Instructions:
7. Preheat waffle iron until hot.
8. In a medium bowl, beat all ingredients except cheese. Stir the jicama mixture into the eggs.
9. Place 1 tablespoon grated cheese on that waffle iron.
10. Spoon 2 heaping tablespoons of the egg/jicama mixture into the waffle iron and top with another tablespoon cheese.
11. Close the waffle maker and cook 5-7

minutes until nicely browned and crunchy.
12. Remove to a wire rack.
13. Repeat 3-4 times.
14. Keto Apple Fritter Chaffle Icing Instructions:
15. Melt butter in a small saucepan and add the Swerve and heavy cream.
16. Simmer over medium heat for 5 minutes or until slightly thickened.
17. Stir in vanilla.
18. Drizzle the hot icing over the chaffles. It will harden as it cools.

151. Monte Cristo Chaffle Crepes Recipe

Preparation time: 15 minutes
Cooking time: 5 minutes
Servings: 3

Ingredients:

- 1 egg
- 1 T almond flour
- 1/4 tsp vanilla extract
- 1/2 T Swerve Confectioners
- 1 T cream cheese softened
- 1 tsp heavy cream
- Pinch of cinnamon

Directions:

1. Mix all ingredients in a small blender.
2. Let batter rest for 5 minutes.
3. Pour 1 1/2 Tablespoons of batter in preheated dash griddle.
4. Cook 30 seconds.
5. Flip with tongs and cook a few more seconds.
6. Place 1 slice of cheese, 1 slice of ham

and 1 slice of turkey on each crepe.

7. If desired, microwave for a few seconds to slightly melt the cheese.

8. Roll the crepes with the filling on the inside.

9. Serve the filled crepes sprinkled with Swerve Confectioners and drizzled with low carb raspberry jam.

152. Easy Turkey Burger with Halloumi Cheese Chaffle Recipe

Preparation time: 10 minutes
Cooking time: 7 minutes
Servings 4

Ingredients:

- 1 lb Ground Turkey raw (no need to precook the turkey)
- 8 oz Halloumi shredded
- 1 zucchini medium, shredded
- 2 tbsp Chives chopped
- 1/2 tsp Salt
- 1/4 tsp Pepper

Directions:

1. Add all ingredients to a bowl mix thoroughly together.

2. Shape into 8 evenly sized patties

3. Preheat mini griddle.

4. Cook the patties for 5-7 minutes.

153. Chaffles with Keto Ice Cream

Preparation Time: 10 minutes
Cooking Time: 14 minutes
Servings: 2

Ingredients:

- 1 egg, beaten
- ½ cup finely grated mozzarella cheese

- ¼ cup almond flour
- 2 tbsp swerve confectioner's sugar
- 1/8 tsp xanthan gum
- Low-carb ice cream (flavor of your choice) for serving

Directions:

1. Preheat the waffle iron.

2. In a medium bowl, mix all the ingredients except the ice cream.

3. Open the iron and add half of the mixture. Close and cook until crispy, 7 minutes.

4. Transfer the chaffle to a plate and make second one with the remaining batter.

5. On each chaffle, add a scoop of low carb ice cream, fold into half-moons and enjoy.

154. Chaffled Brownie Sundae

Preparation Time: 12 minutes
Cooking Time: 30 minutes
Servings: 4

Ingredients:

- For the chaffles:
- 2 eggs, beaten
- 1 tbsp unsweetened cocoa powder
- 1 tbsp erythritol
- 1 cup finely grated mozzarella cheese
- For the topping:
- 3 tbsp unsweetened chocolate, chopped
- 3 tbsp unsalted butter
- ½ cup swerve sugar
- Low-carb ice cream for topping
- 1 cup whipped cream for topping

- 3 tbsp sugar-free caramel sauce

Directions:

1. For the chaffles:
2. Preheat the waffle iron.
3. Meanwhile, in a medium bowl, mix all the ingredients for the chaffles.
4. Open the iron, pour in a quarter of the mixture, cover, and cook until crispy, 7 minutes.
5. Remove the chaffle onto a plate and make 3 more with the remaining batter.
6. Plate and set aside.
7. For the topping:
8. Meanwhile, melt the chocolate and butter in a medium saucepan with occasional stirring, 2 minutes.
9. To Servings:
10. Divide the chaffles into wedges and top with the ice cream, whipped cream, and swirl the chocolate sauce and caramel sauce on top.
11. Serve immediately.

155.Italian Sausage Chaffles

Preparation Time: 5 minutes
Cooking Time: 8 minutes
Servings: 2

Ingredients:

- 1 egg, beaten
- 1 cup cheddar cheese, shredded
- ¼ cup Parmesan cheese, grated
- 1 lb. Italian sausage, crumbled
- 2 teaspoons baking powder
- 1 cup almond flour

Directions:

1. Preheat your waffle maker.

2. Mix all the ingredients in a bowl.
3. Pour half of the mixture into the waffle maker.
4. Cover and cook for 4 minutes.
5. Transfer to a plate.
6. Let cool to make it crispy.
7. Do the same steps to make the next chaffle.

156.Keto Icecream Chaffle

Preparation Time: 15 minutes
Cooking Time: 15 minutes
Servings: 2

Ingredients:

- Egg: 1
- Swerve/Monkfruit: 2 tbsp
- Baking powder: 1 tbsp
- Heavy whipping cream: 1 tbsp
- Keto ice cream: as per your choice

Directions:

1. Take a small bowl and whisk the egg and add all the ingredients
2. Beat until the mixture becomes creamy
3. Pour the mixture to the lower plate of the waffle maker and spread it evenly to cover the plate properly
4. Close the lid
5. Cook for at least 4 minutes to get the desired crunch
6. Remove the chaffle from the heat and keep aside for a few minutes
7. Make as many chaffles as your mixture and waffle maker allow
8. Top with your favorite ice cream and enjoy!

157.Double Chocolate Chaffle

Preparation Time: 5 minutes
Cooking Time: 10 minutes
Servings: 2

Ingredients:

- Egg: 2
- Coconut flour: 4 tbsp
- Cocoa powder: 2 tbsp
- Cream cheese: 2 oz
- Baking powder: ½ tsp
- Chocolate chips: 2 tbsp (unsweetened)
- Vanilla extract: 1 tsp
- Swerve/Monkfruit: 4 tbsp

Directions:

1. Preheat a mini waffle maker if needed and grease it
2. In a mixing bowl, beat eggs
3. In a separate mixing bowl, add coconut flour, cocoa powder, Swerve/Monkfruit, and baking powder, when combine pour into eggs with cream cheese and vanilla extracts
4. Mix them all well to give them uniform consistency and pour the mixture to the lower plate of the waffle maker
5. On top of the mixture, sprinkle around half tsp of unsweetened chocolate chips and close the lid
6. Cook for at least 4 minutes to get the desired crunch
7. Remove the chaffle from the heat and keep aside for around one minute
8. Make as many chaffles as your mixture and waffle maker allow
9. Serve with your favorite whipped cream or berries

158.Cream Cheese Mini Chaffle

Preparation Time: 5 minutes
Cooking Time: 10 minutes
Servings: 2

Ingredients:

- Egg: 1
- Coconut flour: 2 tbsp
- Cream cheese: 1 oz
- Baking powder: ¼ tsp
- Vanilla extract: ½ tsp
- Swerve/Monkfruit: 4 tsp

Directions:

1. Preheat a waffle maker if needed and grease it
2. In a mixing bowl, mix coconut flour, Swerve/Monkfruit, and baking powder
3. Now add an egg to the mixture with cream cheese and vanilla extract
4. Mix them all well and pour the mixture to the lower plate of the waffle maker
5. Close the lid
6. Cook for at least 4 minutes to get the desired crunch
7. Remove the chaffle from the heat
8. Make as many chaffles as your mixture and waffle maker allow
9. Eat the chaffles with your favorite toppings

159.Blackberries Chaffle

Preparation Time: 15 minutes
Cooking Time: 20 minutes
Servings: 4

Ingredients:

- Cheddar cheese: 1/3 cup
- Egg: 1
- Blackberries: 1/2 cup
- Almond flour: 2 tbsp
- Baking powder: 1/4 teaspoon
- Ground almonds: 2 tbsp
- Mozzarella cheese: 1/3 cup

Directions:

1. Mix cheddar cheese, egg, blackberries, almond flour, almond ground, and baking powder together in a bowl
2. Preheat your waffle iron and grease it
3. In your mini waffle iron, shred half of the mozzarella cheese
4. Add the mixture to your mini waffle iron
5. Again shred the remaining mozzarella cheese on the mixture
6. Cook till the desired crisp is achieved
7. Make as many chaffles as your mixture and waffle maker allow

160.Choco Chip Cannoli Chaffle

Preparation Time: 10 minutes
Cooking Time: 20 minutes
Servings: 4

Ingredients:

- For Chaffle:
- Egg yolk: 1
- Swerve/Monkfruit: 1 tbsp
- Baking powder: 1/8 tbsp
- Vanilla extract: 1/8 tsp
- Almond flour: 3 tbsp
- Chocolate chips: 1 tbsp

- For Cannoli Topping:
- Cream cheese: 4 tbsp
- Ricotta: 6 tbsp
- Sweetener: 2 tbsp
- Vanilla extract: ¼ tbsp
- Lemon extract: 5 drops

Directions:

1. Preheat a mini waffle maker if needed and grease it
2. In a mixing bowl, add all the chaffle ingredients and mix well
3. Pour the mixture to the lower plate of the waffle maker and spread it evenly to cover the plate properly and close the lid
4. Cook for at least 4 minutes to get the desired crunch
5. In the meanwhile, prepare cannoli topping by adding all the ingredients in the blender to give the creamy texture
6. Remove the chaffle from the heat and keep aside to cool them down
7. Make as many chaffles as your mixture and waffle maker allow
8. Serve with the cannoli toppings and enjoy

161.Coco Cinnamon Chaffles

Preparation Time: 5 minutes
Cooking Time: 20 minutes
Servings: 4

Ingredients:

- Cheddar cheese: 1/3 cup
- Egg: 1
- Monkfruit sweetener: 1 tsp
- Cinnamon powder: 2 tbsp

- Coconut flour: 2 tbsp
- Baking powder: 1/4 teaspoon
- Coconut flakes: 2 tbsp
- Mozzarella cheese: 1/3 cup

Directions:

1. Mix cheddar cheese, egg, coconut flour, coconut flakes, monk fruit sweetener, and baking powder together in a bowl
2. Preheat your waffle iron and grease it
3. In your mini waffle iron, shred half of the mozzarella cheese
4. Add the mixture to your mini waffle iron
5. Again shred the remaining mozzarella cheese on the mixture
6. Cook till the desired crisp is achieved
7. Make as many chaffles as your mixture and waffle maker allow
8. Sprinkle cinnamon powder on top

162.Tomato Onions Chaffles

Preparation Time: 10 minutes
Cooking Time: 20 minutes
Servings: 2

Ingredients:

- For the Chaffle:
- Egg: 1
- Mozzarella Cheese: 1/2 cup (shredded)
- Onion: ½ cup chopped
- Garlic powder: ½ tsp
- Dried basil: ½ tsp
- For Baking:
- Tomato: 1 large thickly sliced
- Mozzarella cheese: ½ cup (shredded)

- Oregano: ½ tsp

Directions:

1. Preheat a mini waffle maker if needed and grease it
2. In a mixing bowl, add all the ingredients of the chaffle and mix well
3. Pour the mixture to the waffle maker
4. Cook for at least 4 minutes to get the desired crunch and make as many chaffles as your batter allows
5. Preheat the oven
6. Spread chaffles on the baking sheet and top one tomato slice
7. Sprinkle cheese on top and put the baking sheet into the oven
8. Heat for 5 minutes to melt the cheese
9. Spread oregano on top and serve hot

163.Cream Cheese Pumpkin Chaffle

Preparation Time: 5 minutes
Cooking Time: 10 minutes
Servings: 2

Ingredients:

- Egg: 2
- Cream cheese: 2 oz
- Coconut flour: 2 tsp
- Swerve/Monkfruit: 4 tsp
- Baking powder: ½ tsp
- Vanilla extract: 1 tsp
- Canned pumpkin: 2 tbsp
- Pumpkin spice: ½ tsp

Directions:

1. Take a small mixing bowl and add Swerve/Monkfruit, coconut flour, and baking powder and mix them all well
2. Now add egg, vanilla extract,

pumpkin, and cream cheese, and beat them all together till uniform consistency is achieved

3. Preheat a mini waffle maker if needed

4. Pour the mixture to the greasy waffle maker

5. Cook for at least 4 minutes to get the desired crunch

6. Remove the chaffle from the heat

7. Make as many chaffles as your mixture and waffle maker allow

8. Serve with butter or whipped cream that you like!

164.Berries –Coco Chaffles

Preparation Time: 5 minutes
Cooking Time: 20 minutes
Servings: 4

Ingredients:

- Cheddar cheese: 1/3 cup
- Egg: 1
- Blackberries: ½ cup
- Coconut flour: 2 tbsp
- Baking powder: 1/4 teaspoon
- Coconut flakes: 2 tbsp
- Mozzarella cheese: 1/3 cup

Directions:

1. Mix cheddar cheese, egg, coconut flour, coconut flakes, blackberries, and baking powder together in a bowl

2. Preheat your waffle iron and grease it

3. In your mini waffle iron, shred half of the mozzarella cheese

4. Add the mixture to your mini waffle iron

5. Again shred the remaining mozzarella cheese on the mixture

6. Cook till the desired crisp is achieved

7. Make as many chaffles as your mixture and waffle maker allow

165.Plum and Almonds Chaffle

Preparation Time: 15 minutes
Cooking Time: 20 minutes
Servings: 4

Ingredients:

- Cheddar cheese: 1/3 cup
- Egg: 1
- Lemon juice: 1 tbsp
- Plum: ½ cup puree
- Almond flour: 2 tbsp
- Baking powder: 1/4 teaspoon
- Ground almonds: 2 tbsp
- Mozzarella cheese: 1/3 cup

Directions:

1. Mix cheddar cheese, egg, lemon juice, almond flour, plum, almond ground, and baking powder together in a bowl

2. Preheat your waffle iron and grease it

3. In your mini waffle iron, shred half of the mozzarella cheese

4. Add the mixture to your mini waffle iron

5. Again shred the remaining mozzarella cheese on the mixture

6. Cook till the desired crisp is achieved

7. Make as many chaffles as your mixture and waffle

166.Easy Blueberry Chaffle

Preparation Time: 5 minutes
Cooking Time: 10 minutes
Servings: 2

Ingredients:

- Egg: 2
- Cream cheese: 2 oz
- Coconut flour: 2 tbsp
- Swerve/Monkfruit: 4 tsp
- Baking powder: ½ tsp
- Vanilla extract: 1 tsp
- Blueberries: ½ cup

Directions:

1. Take a small mixing bowl and add Swerve/Monkfruit, baking powder, and coconut flour and mix them all well

2. Now add eggs, vanilla extract, and cream cheese, and beat them all together till uniform consistency is achieved

3. Preheat a mini waffle maker if needed and grease it

4. Pour the mixture to the lower plate of the waffle maker

5. Add 3-4 fresh blueberries above the mixture and close the lid

6. Cook for at least 4 minutes to get the desired crunch

7. Remove the chaffle from the heat

8. Make as many chaffles as your mixture and waffle maker allow

9. Serve with butter or whipped cream that you like!

167. Sweet and Sour Coconut Chaffles

Preparation Time: 5 minutes
Cooking Time: 20 minutes
Servings: 4

Ingredients:

- Cheddar cheese: 1/3 cup
- Egg: 1
- Monkfruit sweetener: 2 tsp
- Lemon juice: 2 tbsp
- Coconut flour: 2 tbsp
- Baking powder: 1/4 teaspoon
- Coconut flakes: 2 tbsp
- Mozzarella cheese: 1/3 cup

Directions:

1. Mix cheddar cheese, egg, coconut flour, coconut flakes, monkfruit sweetener, lemon juice, and baking powder together in a bowl

2. Preheat your waffle iron and grease it

3. In your mini waffle iron, shred half of the mozzarella cheese

4. Add the mixture to your mini waffle iron

5. Again shred the remaining mozzarella cheese on the mixture

6. Cook till the desired crisp is achieved

7. Make as many chaffles as your mixture and waffle maker allow

8. Sprinkle cinnamon powder on top

168. Plum Coconut Chaffles

Preparation Time: 5 minutes
Cooking Time: 20 minutes
Servings: 4

Ingredients:

- Cheddar cheese: 1/3 cup
- Egg: 1
- Plum: ½ cup pureed
- Coconut flour: 2 tbsp
- Baking powder: 1/4 teaspoon
- Coconut flakes: 2 tbsp
- Mozzarella cheese: 1/3 cup

Directions:

1. Mix cheddar cheese, egg, coconut flour, coconut flakes, plum puree, and baking powder together in a bowl

2. Preheat your waffle iron and grease it

3. In your mini waffle iron, shred half of the mozzarella cheese

4. Add the mixture to your mini waffle iron

5. Again shred the remaining mozzarella cheese on the mixture

6. Cook till the desired crisp is achieved

7. Make as many chaffles as your mixture and waffle maker allow

169.Apple Pie Chayote Tacos Chaffle

Preparation Time: 15 minutes
Cooking Time: 50 minutes
Servings: 2
Ingredients:

- For Chaffle:
- Egg: 2
- Cream cheese: ½ cup
- Baking powder: 1 tsp
- Vanilla extract: ½ tsp
- Powdered sweetener: 2 tbsp
- For Apple Pie Chayote Filling:
- Chayote squash: 1
- Butter: 1 tbsp
- Swerve: ¼ cup
- Cinnamon powder: 2 tsp
- Lemon: 2 tbsp
- Cream of tartar: 1/8 tsp
- Nutmeg: 1/8 tsp
- Ginger powder: 1/8 tsp

Directions:

1. For around 25 minutes, boil the whole chayote; when it cools, peel it and slice

2. Add all the remaining filling ingredients to it

3. Bake the chayote for 20 minutes covered with foil

4. Pour ¼ of the mixtures to the blender to make it a sauce

5. Add to chayote slices and mix

6. For the chaffles, preheat a mini waffle maker if needed and grease it

7. In a mixing bowl, add all the chaffle ingredients and mix well

8. Pour the mixture to the lower plate of the waffle maker and spread it evenly to cover the plate properly and close the lid

9. Cook for at least 4 minutes to get the desired crunch

10. Make as many chaffles as your mixture and waffle maker allow

11. Fold the chaffles and serve with the chayote sauce in between

170.Kiwi Almonds Chaffle

Preparation Time: 15 minutes
Cooking Time: 20 minutes
Servings: 4

Ingredients:

- Cheddar cheese: 1/3 cup
- Egg: 1
- Kiwi: ½ cup mashed
- Almond flour: 2 tbsp
- Baking powder: 1/4 teaspoon
- Ground almonds: 2 tbsp
- Mozzarella cheese: 1/3 cup

Directions:

1. Mix cheddar cheese, egg, lemon juice, almond flour, kiwi, almond ground, and baking powder together in a bowl

2. Preheat your waffle iron and grease it

3. In your mini waffle iron, shred half of the mozzarella cheese

4. Add the mixture to your mini waffle iron

5. Again shred the remaining mozzarella cheese on the mixture

6. Cook till the desired crisp is achieved

7. Make as many chaffles as your mixture and waffle maker allow

171.Rice Krispie Treat Copycat Chaffle

Preparation Time: 15 minutes
Cooking Time: 25 minutes
Servings: 2

Ingredients:

- For Chaffle:
- Egg: 1
- Cream cheese: 4 tbsp
- Baking powder: 1 tsp
- Vanilla extract: ½ tsp
- Powdered sweetener: 2 tbsp
- Pork rinds: 4 tbsp (crushed)
- For Marshmallow Frosting:
- Heavy whipping cream: ¼ cup
- Xanthan gum: ½ tsp
- Powdered sweetener: 1 tbsp
- Vanilla extract: ¼ tsp

Directions:

1. Preheat a mini waffle maker if needed and grease it

2. In a mixing bowl, add all the chaffle ingredients

3. Mix them all well

4. Pour the mixture to the lower plate of the waffle maker and spread it evenly to cover the plate properly and close the lid

5. Cook for at least 4 minutes to get the desired crunch

6. Remove the chaffle from the heat and keep aside for around one minute

7. Make as many chaffles as your mixture and waffle maker allow

8. For the marshmallow frosting, add all the frosting ingredients except xanthan gum and whip to form a thick consistency

9. Add xanthan gum at the end and fold

10. Serve frosting with chaffles and enjoy!

172.Peppermint Mocha Chaffle

Preparation Time: 10 minutes
Cooking Time: 20 minutes
Servings: 2

Ingredients:

- For Chaffle:
- Egg: 1
- Powdered sweetener: 2 tbsp
- Cream cheese: 2 tbsp
- Butter: 2 tbsp (melted)
- Coconut flour: 2 tsp
- Almond flour: 1 tsp
- Baking powder: 1/4 tsp
- Vanilla extract: ¼ tsp
- Cocoa powder: 1 tbsp (unsweetened)
- Salt: a pinch
- For Filling:
- Butter: 2 tbsp

- Heavy cream: ½ cup
- Powdered sweetener: 2 tbsp
- Vanilla extract: ¼ tsp
- Peppermint extract: 1/8 tsp
- Starlight mints: for garnishing

Directions:

1. Preheat a mini waffle maker if needed and grease it
2. In a mixing bowl, add all the chaffle ingredients
3. Mix them all well
4. Pour the mixture to the lower plate of the waffle maker and spread it evenly to cover the plate properly and close the lid
5. Cook for at least 4 minutes to get the desired crunch
6. Remove the chaffle from the heat and keep aside for around one minute
7. Make as many chaffles as your mixture and waffle maker allow
8. For the filling, add all the filling ingredients and beat at high speed using the hand blender
9. On each chaffle spread the filling and top with starlight mint

173.Coco-Kiwi Chaffles

Preparation Time: 5 minutes
Cooking Time: 20 minutes
Servings: 4

Ingredients:

- Cheddar cheese: 1/3 cup
- Egg: 1
- Kiwi: ½ cup finely grated
- Coconut flour: 2 tbsp
- Baking powder: 1/4 teaspoon

- Coconut flakes: 2 tbsp
- Mozzarella cheese: 1/3 cup

Directions:

1. Mix cheddar cheese, egg, coconut flour, coconut flakes, kiwi, and baking powder together in a bowl
2. Preheat your waffle iron and grease it
3. In your mini waffle iron, shred half of the mozzarella cheese
4. Add the mixture to your mini waffle iron
5. Again shred the remaining mozzarella cheese on the mixture
6. Cook till the desired crisp is achieved
7. Make as many chaffles as your mixture and waffle maker allow

174.Rhubarb Almonds Chaffle

Preparation Time: 15 minutes
Cooking Time: 20 minutes
Servings: 4

Ingredients:

- Cheddar cheese: 1/3 cup
- Egg: 1
- Rhubarb puree: 1/4 cup
- Almond flour: 2 tbsp
- Baking powder: 1/4 teaspoon
- Ground almonds: 2 tbsp
- Mozzarella cheese: 1/3 cup

Directions:

1. Mix cheddar cheese, egg, rhubarb puree, almond flour, almond ground, and baking powder together in a bowl
2. Preheat your waffle iron and grease it
3. In your mini waffle iron, shred half of the mozzarella cheese

4. Add the mixture to your mini waffle iron

5. Again shred the remaining mozzarella cheese on the mixture

6. Cook till the desired crisp is achieved

7. Make as many chaffles as your mixture and waffle maker allow

175.Strawberry Coconut Chaffles

Preparation Time: 5 minutes
Cooking Time: 20 minutes
Servings: 4

Ingredients:

- Cheddar cheese: 1/3 cup
- Egg: 1
- Strawberry: ½ cup finely chopped or mashed
- Coconut flour: 2 tbsp
- Baking powder: 1/4 teaspoon
- Coconut flakes: 2 tbsp
- Mozzarella cheese: 1/3 cup

Directions:

1. Mix cheddar cheese, egg, coconut flour, coconut flakes, strawberry, and baking powder together in a bowl

2. Preheat your waffle iron and grease it

3. In your mini waffle iron, shred half of the mozzarella cheese

4. Add the mixture to your mini waffle iron

5. Again shred the remaining mozzarella cheese on the mixture

6. Cook till the desired crisp is achieved

7. Make as many chaffles as your mixture and waffle maker allow

176.Almonds and Raspberries Chaffles

Preparation Time: 15 minutes
Cooking Time: 20 minutes
Servings: 4

What You Need:

- Cheddar cheese: 1/3 cup
- Egg: 1
- Raspberries: ½ cup
- Almond flour: 2 tbsp
- Baking powder: 1/4 teaspoon
- Ground almonds: 2 tbsp
- Mozzarella cheese: 1/3 cup

Directions:

1. Mix cheddar cheese, egg, raspberries, almond flour, almond ground, and baking powder together in a bowl

2. Preheat your waffle iron and grease it

3. In your mini waffle iron, shred half of the mozzarella cheese

4. Add the mixture to your mini waffle iron

5. Again shred the remaining mozzarella cheese on the mixture

6. Cook till the desired crisp is achieved

7. Make as many chaffles as your mixture and waffle maker allow

177.Churro Chaffle

Preparation Time: 5 minutes
Cooking Time: 10 minutes
Servings: 2

Ingredients:

- Egg: 2
- Mozzarella Cheese: 1 cup (shredded)
- Swerve Brown sweetener: 4 tbsp
- Cinnamon powder: 1 tsp

Directions:

1. Preheat a mini waffle maker if needed and grease it

2. In a mixing bowl, beat eggs and add cheese to them

3. Mix them all well and pour the mixture to the lower plate of the waffle maker

4. Close the lid

5. Cook for at least 4 minutes to get the desired crunch

6. In the meanwhile, mix Swerve Brown sweetener and cinnamon powder in a separate bowl

7. Remove the chaffle from the heat and cut it into slices when still hot ad add to the cinnamon mixture

8. Make as many chaffles as your mixture and waffle maker allow

9. Serve hot and enjoy!

178. Crunchy Strawberry Chaffle

Preparation Time: 5 minutes
Cooking Time: 10 minutes
Servings: 2

Ingredients:

- Egg: 2
- Cream cheese: 2 tbsp
- Mozzarella Cheese: ½ cup
- Baking powder: ½ tsp
- Whipping cream: 2 tbsp
- Strawberry: 4
- Strawberry extract: 2 tsp

Directions:

1. Preheat a mini waffle maker if needed and grease it

2. In a mixing bowl, beat eggs and add mozzarella cheese to them

3. Now add strawberry extract, cream cheese, and baking powder

4. Mix them all well and pour the mixture to the lower plate of the waffle maker

5. Close the lid

6. Cook for at least 5 minutes to get the desired crunch

7. Remove the chaffle from the heat and keep aside for around one minute

8. Make as many chaffles as your mixture and waffle maker allow

9. Serve with whipped cream and sliced strawberries on top

179. Fresh Strawberries Chaffle

Preparation Time: 5 minutes
Cooking Time: 10 minutes
Servings: 2

Ingredients:

- Egg: 1
- Mozzarella Cheese: ½ cup
- Almond flour: 1 tbsp
- Swerve: 1½ tbsp
- Vanilla extract: ¼ tsp
- Whipped cream: 2 tbsp
- Strawberry: 4

Directions:

1. Preheat a mini waffle maker if needed

2. Chop fresh strawberries and mix with half tablespoon of granulated swerve and keep it aside

3. In a mixing bowl, beat eggs and add mozzarella cheese, almond flour, granulated swerve, and vanilla extract

4. Mix them all well and pour the mixture to the lower plate of the waffle maker

5. Close the lid

6. Cook for at least 4 minutes to get the desired crunch

7. Remove the chaffle from the heat and keep aside for around two minute

8. Make as many chaffles as your mixture and waffle maker allow

9. Serve with the fresh strawberries mixture you made with the whipped cream on top

180. Chocolate Melt Chaffles

Preparation Time: 15 minutes
Cooking Time: 36 minutes
Servings: 4

Ingredients

- For the chaffles:
- 2 eggs, beaten
- ¼ cup finely grated Gruyere cheese
- 2 tbsp heavy cream
- 1 tbsp coconut flour
- 2 tbsp cream cheese, softened
- 3 tbsp unsweetened cocoa powder
- 2 tsp vanilla extract
- A pinch of salt
- For the chocolate sauce:
- 1/3 cup + 1 tbsp heavy cream
- 1 ½ oz unsweetened baking chocolate, chopped
- 1 ½ tsp sugar-free maple syrup
- 1 ½ tsp vanilla extract

Directions:

1. For the chaffles:

2. Preheat the waffle iron.

3. In a medium bowl, mix all the ingredients for the chaffles.

4. Open the iron and add a quarter of the mixture. Close and cook until crispy, 7 minutes.

5. Transfer the chaffle to a plate and make 3 more with the remaining batter.

6. For the chocolate sauce:

7. Pour the heavy cream into saucepan and simmer over low heat, 3 minutes.

8. Turn the heat off and add the chocolate. Allow melting for a few minutes and stir until fully melted, 5 minutes.

9. Mix in the maple syrup and vanilla extract.

10. Assemble the chaffles in layers with the chocolate sauce sandwiched between each layer.

11. Slice and serve immediately.

181. Strawberry Shortcake Chaffle Bowls

Preparation Time: 10 minutes
Cooking Time: 28 minutes
Servings: 4
Ingredients:

- 1 egg, beaten
- ½ cup finely grated mozzarella cheese
- 1 tbsp almond flour
- ¼ tsp baking powder
- 2 drops cake batter extract
- 1 cup cream cheese, softened
- 1 cup fresh strawberries, sliced
- 1 tbsp sugar-free maple syrup

Directions:

1. Preheat a waffle bowl maker and grease lightly with cooking spray.

2. Meanwhile, in a medium bowl, whisk all the ingredients except the cream

cheese and strawberries.

3. Open the iron, pour in half of the mixture, cover, and cook until crispy, 6 to 7 minutes.

4. Remove the chaffle bowl onto a plate and set aside.

5. Make a second chaffle bowl with the remaining batter.

6. To serve, divide the cream cheese into the chaffle bowls and top with the strawberries.

7. Drizzle the filling with the maple syrup and serve.

182.Chaffles with Raspberry Syrup

Preparation Time: 10 minutes
Cooking Time: 38 minutes
Servings: 4

Ingredients:

- For the chaffles:
- 1 egg, beaten
- ½ cup finely shredded cheddar cheese
- 1 tsp almond flour
- 1 tsp sour cream
- For the raspberry syrup:
- 1 cup fresh raspberries
- ¼ cup swerve sugar
- ¼ cup water
- 1 tsp vanilla extract

Directions:

1. For the chaffles:
2. Preheat the waffle iron.
3. Meanwhile, in a medium bowl, mix the egg, cheddar cheese, almond flour, and sour cream.
4. Open the iron, pour in half of the mixture, cover, and cook until crispy,

7 minutes.

5. Remove the chaffle onto a plate and make another with the remaining batter.

6. For the raspberry syrup:

7. Meanwhile, add the raspberries, swerve sugar, water, and vanilla extract to a medium pot. Set over low heat and cook until the raspberries soften and sugar becomes syrupy. Occasionally stir while mashing the raspberries as you go. Turn the heat off when your desired consistency is achieved and set aside to cool.

8. Drizzle some syrup on the chaffles and enjoy when ready.

183.Chaffle Cannoli

Preparation Time: 15 minutes
Cooking Time: 28 minutes
Servings: 4

Ingredients:

- For the chaffles:
- 1 large egg
- 1 egg yolk
- 3 tbsp butter, melted
- 1 tbso swerve confectioner's
- 1 cup finely grated Parmesan cheese
- 2 tbsp finely grated mozzarella cheese
- For the cannoli filling:
- ½ cup ricotta cheese
- 2 tbsp swerve confectioner's sugar
- 1 tsp vanilla extract
- 2 tbsp unsweetened chocolate chips for garnishing

Directions:

1. Preheat the waffle iron.

2. Meanwhile, in a medium bowl, mix all the ingredients for the chaffles.

3. Open the iron, pour in a quarter of the mixture, cover, and cook until crispy, 7 minutes.

4. Remove the chaffle onto a plate and make 3 more with the remaining batter.

5. Meanwhile, for the cannoli filling:

6. Beat the ricotta cheese and swerve confectioner's sugar until smooth. Mix in the vanilla.

7. On each chaffle, spread some of the filling and wrap over.

8. Garnish the creamy ends with some chocolate chips.

9. Serve immediately.

184.Blueberry Chaffles

Preparation Time: 10 minutes
Cooking Time: 28 minutes
Servings: 4

Ingredients:

- 1 egg, beaten
- ½ cup finely grated mozzarella cheese
- 1 tbsp cream cheese, softened
- 1 tbsp sugar-free maple syrup + extra for topping
- ½ cup blueberries
- ¼ tsp vanilla extract

Directions:

1. Preheat the waffle iron.

2. In a medium bowl, mix all the ingredients.

3. Open the iron, lightly grease with cooking spray and pour in a quarter of the mixture.

4. Close the iron and cook until golden

brown and crispy, 7 minutes.

5. Remove the chaffle onto a plate and set aside.

6. Make the remaining chaffles with the remaining mixture.

7. Drizzle the chaffles with maple syrup and serve afterward.

185.Nutter Butter Chaffles

Preparation Time: 15 minutes
Cooking Time: 14 minutes
Servings: 2

Ingredients:

- For the chaffles:
- 2 tbsp sugar-free peanut butter powder
- 2 tbsp maple (sugar-free) syrup
- 1 egg, beaten
- ¼ cup finely grated mozzarella cheese
- ¼ tsp baking powder
- ¼ tsp almond butter
- ¼ tsp peanut butter extract
- 1 tbsp softened cream cheese
- For the frosting:
- ½ cup almond flour
- 1 cup peanut butter
- 3 tbsp almond milk
- ½ tsp vanilla extract
- ½ cup maple (sugar-free) syrup

Directions:

1. Preheat the waffle iron.

2. Meanwhile, in a medium bowl, mix all the ingredients until smooth.

3. Open the iron and pour in half of the mixture.

4. Close the iron and cook until crispy, 6 to 7 minutes.

5. Remove the chaffle onto a plate and set aside.

6. Make a second chaffle with the remaining batter.

7. While the chaffles cool, make the frosting.

8. Pour the almond flour in a medium saucepan and stir-fry over medium heat until golden.

9. Transfer the almond flour to a blender and top with the remaining frosting ingredients. Process until smooth.

10. Spread the frosting on the chaffles and serve afterward.

186.Brie and Blackberry Chaffles

Preparation Time: 15 minutes
Cooking Time: 36 minutes
Servings: 4

Ingredients:

- For the chaffles:
- 2 eggs, beaten
- 1 cup finely grated mozzarella cheese
- For the topping:
- 1 ½ cups blackberries
- 1 lemon, 1 tsp zest and 2 tbsp juice
- 1 tbsp erythritol
- 4 slices Brie cheese

Directions:

1. For the chaffles:

2. Preheat the waffle iron.

3. Meanwhile, in a medium bowl, mix the eggs and mozzarella cheese.

4. Open the iron, pour in a quarter of the mixture, cover, and cook until crispy, 7 minutes.

5. Remove the chaffle onto a plate and make 3 more with the remaining batter.

6. Plate and set aside.

7. For the topping:

8. Preheat the oven to 350 F and line a baking sheet with parchment paper.

9. In a medium pot, add the blackberries, lemon zest, lemon juice, and erythritol. Cook until the blackberries break and the sauce thickens, 5 minutes. Turn the heat off.

10. Arrange the chaffles on the baking sheet and place two Brie cheese slices on each. Top with blackberry mixture and transfer the baking sheet to the oven.

11. Bake until the cheese melts, 2 to 3 minutes.

12. Remove from the oven, allow cooling and serve afterward.

187.Churro Chaffle

Preparation Time: 4 min
Cooking Time: 5 min
Number of Servings: 2

Ingredients

- 2 eggs
- 1 cup mozzarella cheese, shredded
- 4 tbsp swerve sweetener
- 1 tsp cinnamon

Directions:

1. Preheat your waffle iron.

2. Whisk the eggs with a fork in a bowl. Add in the shredded cheese.

3. Pour half of the egg and cheese mixture into the waffle maker. Cook for 5 minutes or until golden brown.

4. In the meantime, add the cinnamon and the sweetener in a separate bowl.

5. By now, the chaffle is ready. Cut into slices and dip them into the cinnamon mixture while.

6. Serve and enjoy!

188.Churro Waffles

Preparation Time: 5 min
Cooking Time: 10 min
Servings: 1

Ingredients

- 1 tbsp coconut cream
- 1 egg
- 6 tbsp almond flour
- ¼ tsp xanthan gum
- ½ tsp cinnamon
- 2 tbsp keto brown sugar
- Coating:
- 2 tbsp butter, melt
- 1 tbsp keto brown sugar

Directions:

1. Add all the waffle ingredients in a small bowl and mix until thick and sticky.

2. Warm up your waffle maker.

3. Pour half of the batter to the waffle pan and cook for 5 minutes.

4. Carefully remove the cooked waffle and repeat the steps with the remaining batter.

5. Allow the chaffles to cool and spread with the melted butter and top with the brown sugar.

6. Enjoy.

189.Ube Chaffles with Ice Cream

Preparation Time: 4 min
Cooking Time: 10 min
Servings: 2

Ingredients

- 1/3 cup mozzarella cheese, shredded
- 1 tbsp whipped cream cheese
- 2 tbsp sweetener
- 1 egg
- 2-3 drops ube or pandan extract
- 1/2 tsp baking powder
- Keto ice cream

Directions:

1. Preheat your mini waffle maker.

2. Combine together all the ingredients in a small bowl, except ube extract. Mix well.

3. Add in 2 or 3 drops of ube extract, mix until creamy and smooth.

4. Pour half of the batter mixture in the mini waffle maker and cook for about 5 minutes.

5. Repeat the same steps with the remaining batter mixture.

6. Top with keto ice cream and enjoy.

190.Chaffle Glazed with Raspberry

Preparation Time: 7 min
Cooking Time: 5 min
Servings: 1

Ingredients

- Donut Chaffle Ingredients:
- 1 egg
- ¼ cup mozzarella cheese, shredded
- 2 tsp cream cheese, softened
- 1 tsp sweetener
- 1tsp almond flour

- ½ tsp baking powder
- 20 drops glazed donut flavoring
- Raspberry Jelly Filling:
- ¼ cup raspberries
- 1 tsp chia seeds
- 1 tsp confectioners sweetener
- Donut Glaze:
- 1 tsp powdered sweetener
- Heavy whipping cream

Directions:

1. Chaffles:
2. Preheat your waffle maker.
3. Mix all the chaffle ingredients.
4. Spray your waffle maker with cooking oil and add the batter mixture into the waffle maker.
5. Cook for 3 minutes and set aside.
6. Raspberry Jelly Filling:
7. Mix all the ingredients under the filling section.
8. Place in a pot and heat on medium.
9. Gently mash the raspberries and set aside to cool.
10. Donut Glaze:
11. Stir together the ingredients in a small dish.
12. Assembling:
13. Lay your chaffles on a plate and add the fillings mixture between the layers.
14. Drizzle the glaze on top and enjoy.

191.Cream Cake Chaffle

Preparation Time: 7 min
Cooking Time: 12 min
Servings: 4

Ingredients

- Chaffle Ingredients:
- 4 oz cream cheese, softened
- 4 eggs
- 4 tbsp coconut flour
- 1 tbsp almond flour
- 1 ½ tsp baking powder
- 1 tbsp butter, softened
- 1 tsp vanilla extract
- ½ tsp cinnamon
- 1 tbsp sweetener
- 1 tbsp shredded coconut, colored and unsweetened
- 1 tbsp walnuts, chopped
- Italian Cream Frosting Ingredients:
- 2 oz cream cheese, softened
- 2 tbsp butter, room temperature
- 2 tbsp sweetener
- ½ tsp vanilla

Directions:

1. Add the almond flour, coconut flour, eggs, cream cheese, softened butter, vanilla, sweetener, and baking powder in a blender and blend until smooth.
2. Add the walnuts and shredded coconut to the mixture.
3. Blend the ingredients on the high setting until you have a creamy mixture.
4. Preheat your waffle maker and add ¼ of the ingredients.
5. Cook for 3 minutes and repeat the process until you have 4 chaffles.
6. Remove and set aside.
7. In the meantime, start making your

frosting by mixing all the ingredients together.

8. Stir until you have a smooth and creamy mixture.

9. Cool, frost the cake and enjoy.

192.Vanilla Chaffle

Preparation Time: 5 min
Cooking Time: 8 min
Servings: 2

Ingredients

- 2 tbsp butter, softened
- 2 oz cream cheese, softened
- 2 eggs
- ¼ cup almond flour
- 2 tbsp coconut flour
- 1 tsp baking powder
- 1 tsp vanilla extract
- ¼ cup confectioners
- Pinch of pink salt

Directions:

1. Preheat the waffle maker and spray with non-stick cooking spray.

2. Melt the butter and set aside for a minute to cool.

3. Add the eggs into the melted butter and whisk until creamy.

4. Pour in the sweetener, vanilla, extract, and salt. Blend properly.

5. Next add the coconut flour, almond flour, and baking powder. Mix well.

6. Pour into the waffle maker and cook for 4 minutes.

7. Repeat the process with the remaining batter.

8. Remove and set aside to cool.

9. Enjoy.

193.Cinnamon Sugar Chaffles

Preparation Time: 7 min
Cooking Time: 12 min
Servings: 2

Ingredients

- 2 eggs
- 1 cup Mozzarella cheese, shredded
- 2 tbsp blanched almond flour
- ½ tbsp butter, melted
- 2 tbsp Erythritol
- ½ tsp cinnamon
- ½ tsp vanilla extract
- ½ tsp psyllium husk powder, optional
- ¼ tsp baking powder, optional
- 1 tbsp melted butter, for topping
- ¼ cup Erythritol, for topping
- ¾ tsp cinnamon, for topping

Directions:

1. Preheat your waffle iron until hot.

2. In the meantime, heat the cream cheese in a microwave for 30 seconds.

3. Add in all the other remaining ingredients with the exception of toppings.

4. Pour enough batter into the waffle maker and cook for 4 minutes.

5. Once the cooked, carefully remove the chaffle and set aside.

6. Repeat with the remaining batter the same steps.

7. Stir together the cinnamon and erythritol.

8. Finish by brushing your chaffles with the melted butter and then sprinkle with cinnamon sugar.

194.Sugar Cookie Chaffles

Preparation Time: 30 minutes
Cooking Time: 10 minutes
Serving: 1 large chaffles or 2 mini chaffles

Ingredients:

- See Sweet Chaffle Recipe
- Classic White Frosting Ingredients:
- 2 tbsp of butter
- 1 ounce of cream cheese
- 10 drops of capella buttercream flavoring
- 1 tsp of vanilla
- 1 tsp of almond extract
- 2 tbsp powdered monk fruit or sweetener of your choice
- 1-3 drops of food coloring of your choice
- Tools: one mixing bowl, measuring cups and tablespoons, spatula, non-stick cooking spray (or butter), blender, electric beaters, or whisk.

Directions:

1. Preheat mini waffle maker.
2. Mix together all the classic white frosting ingredients EXCEPT the food coloring.
3. Once the frosting ingredients are well mixed, divide into 2-3 small bowls or however many colors you want.
4. In each bowl, drop 1-2 droplets of food coloring and mix into the bowl until the color is consistent. Add more drops if you want the color to be brighter. Put aside in the fridge.
5. Take all of your chaffle ingredients, and mix them in a small bowl together.
6. When the waffle iron is ready, evenly pour the batter into the pan.
7. Use your spatula to make sure the batter is well distributed.
8. Wait until your waffle iron says it's ready to take out.
9. If you are making many servings, preheat your oven to the lowest temperature, like 300 degrees F, and put the chaffles on an oven-safe pan to keep warm while making multiple batches.
10. Take a chaffle and layer on the frosting for desired thickness.

195. Chocolate Chip Cookie Chaffle

Preparation Time: 30 minutes
Cooking Time: 10 minutes
Servings: 1 large chaffles or 2 mini chaffles

Chaffle Ingredients:

- Classic Sweet Chaffle Recipe
- 1/2 cup of Lily's Chocolate Chips
- 1 tsp of cinnamon
- Tools: one mixing bowl, measuring cups and tablespoons, spatula, non-stick cooking spray (or butter), blender, electric beaters, or whisk.

Directions:

1. Mix in chocolate chips and cinnamon to the Classic Sweet Chaffle Recipe.
2. Follow the steps for the Classic Sweet Chaffle Recipe.
3. Enjoy!

196. Gingerbread

Preparation Time: 30 minutes
Cooking Time: 10 minutes
Serving: 1 large chaffles or 2 mini chaffles

Ingredients:

- Classic Sweet Chaffle Recipe
- 1/4 cup of cocoa powder

- 1 tsp of cinnamon
- 2 tsp of ginger powder
- Classic White Frosting Recipe
- Tools: one mixing bowl, measuring cups and tablespoons, spatula, non-stick cooking spray (or butter), blender, electric beaters, or whisk.

Directions:

1. Follow the steps for the Classic White Frosting Recipe and set aside.
2. Mix in cocoa powder, ginger powder, and cinnamon to the Classic Sweet Chaffle Recipe.
3. Follow the steps for the Classic Sweet Chaffle Recipe.
4. Serve the chaffles individually and lather on the frosting to each chaffle.
5. Enjoy!

197.Boston Cream Pie Chaffle

Preparation Time: 30 minutes
Cooking Time: 10 minutes
Serving: 1 large chaffles or 2 mini chaffles

Ingredients:

- Classic Sweet Chaffle Recipe
- Custard Ingredients:
- 1/2 a cup of heavy whipping cream
- 1/2 tsp of vanilla extract
- 1 tbsp of swerve confectioner's sweetener
- 2 egg yokes
- 1/8 tsp of xanthan gum
- Ganache Ingredients:
- 2 tbsp of heavy whipping cream
- 2 tbsp unsweetened baking chocolate bar, chopped
- 1 tbsp swerve confectioner's

sweetener
- Tools: one mixing bowl, measuring cups and tablespoons, spatula, non-stick cooking spray (or butter), blender, electric beaters, or whisk.

Directions:

1. Follow the steps for the Classic White Frosting Recipe and set aside.
2. Mix in cocoa powder, ginger powder, and cinnamon to the Classic Sweet Chaffle Recipe.
3. Follow the steps for the Classic Sweet Chaffle Recipe.
4. Serve the chaffles individually and lather on the frosting to each chaffle.
5. Enjoy!

198.Banana Nut Chaffles

Preparation Time: 30 minutes
Cooking Time: 10 minutes
Serving: 1 large chaffles or 2 mini chaffles

Ingredients:

- Classic Sweet Chaffle Recipe
- 1/2 tsp of banana extract
- 1 tsp of cinnamon
- handful of walnuts or pecan nuts, roughly chopped
- Tools: one mixing bowl, measuring cups and tablespoons, spatula, non-stick cooking spray (or butter), blender, electric beaters, or whisk.

Directions:

1. Take the nuts and roughly chop them into quarter size pieces.
2. Mix in banana extract, half the nuts, and cinnamon to the Classic Sweet Chaffle Recipe.
3. Follow the steps for the Classic Sweet

Chaffle Recipe.

4. Serve the chaffles individually and lather on the Classic White Frosting recipe or the Vanilla Sauce to each chaffle if desired.

5. Sprinkle the rest of the nuts on top of your chaffles.

6. Enjoy!

199.Pecan Pie Chaffle

Preparation Time: 30 minutes
Cooking Time: 10 minutes
Serving: 1 large chaffles or 2 mini chaffles

Ingredients:

Classic Sweet Chaffle Recipe

- 1/4 of a tbsp of blackstrap molasses
- 1 cup of pecans, toasted
- 1 tsp of cinnamon
- Keto Caramel Ingredients:
- 2 tbsp of heavy whipping cream
- 2 tbsp of butter
- 1 tbsp of sukrin gold
- 2 egg yolks, large
- 2 tbsp of cream cheese, softened
- 1/2 teaspoon of maple extract
- 1/2 tsp of vanilla extract
- 1 tsp of cinnamon
- 1 tsp of salt
- Tools: one mixing bowl, measuring cups and tablespoons, spatula, non-stick cooking spray (or butter), baking tray, blender, electric beaters, or whisk.

Directions:

1. Preheat the oven to 350 degrees F.

2. When heated, spread the pecans onto a baking sheet and toast for 15 minutes.

3. Crack the eggs and separate the yolks from the whites, set aside.

4. Take a small saucepan and add in the butter, sweetener, and heavy whipping cream on low heat.

5. Continue whisking until the ingredients begin to break up and are well combined.

6. Take the mixture off the heat.

7. Temper the eggs by pouring 1/2 of the cream mixture into the egg yolks and whisk until combined.

8. Add the cream and egg mixture back into the saucepan and keep stirring.

9. Let simmer until it starts to thicken.

10. Add in salt.

11. Take the mixture off of the heat and allow it to cool.

12. Begin making the chaffles.

13. Take the pecans out of the oven and let cool.

14. Directions for the Chaffles:

15. Follow the steps for the Classic Sweet Chaffle Recipe.

16. Lay out three chaffles and spread the Keto Caramel sauce onto each one followed by the toasted pecans and sandwich on top of each other. Top the stack with the remaining sauce and pecans.

17. Enjoy!

200.Lemon Meringue Chaffle

Preparation Time: 30 minutes
Cooking Time: 10 minutes
Serving: 1 large chaffles or 2 mini chaffles

Ingredients:

- Classic Sweet Chaffle Recipe
- 1/2 tsp of lemon extract
- Lemon Curd Ingredients:
- 3 large eggs
- 1/2 cup powdered Swerve Sweetener
- 1/4 cup freshly squeezed lemon juice
- 2 teaspoons grated lemon zest
- 4 tablespoons butter cut into 3 pieces
- Meringue Topping Ingredients:
- 2 large egg whites at room temperature
- 1/4 tsp cream of tartar
- Pinch salt
- 1/4 cup powdered Swerve Sweetener
- 1/4 cup granulated Swerve Sweetener
- Tools: one mixing bowl, measuring cups and tablespoons, spatula, non-stick cooking spray (or butter), double boiler, baking tray, piping bag, blender, electric beaters, or whisk.

Directions:

1. Preheat the oven to 200 degrees F.
2. Take a baking tray and place parchment paper on it to fully cover the bottom.
3. Crack the eggs and separate the whites from the yolks. Put aside.
4. Juice and zest the lemons. Put aside.
5. Whisk the egg whites with electric beaters on low until they become foamy.
6. Take the lemon juice and pour, increase the hand mixer to high.
7. Whip the mixture until hard peaks form. You should be able to hold the bowl upside down and the mixture won't slide.
8. Slowly add the erythritol and lemon zest, one tablespoon at a time.
9. Once everything is combined, pour the mixture into a piping bag.
10. Squeeze the bag onto the parchment paper for your desired shape and size.
11. Put the tray in the oven and bake for one hour. Then turn the oven off and leave the tray in the oven until it cools completely.
12. Leave them in for 1-2 hours before removing the tray from the oven.
13. Once completely cooled, transfer to a dish.
14. Directions for the Lemon Curd:
15. In a double boiler or a pot of boiling water with a glass bowl on top, heat the bottom pot with water and bring to a simmer.
16. Juice the lemon and zest it until you have enough.
17. Slice off the butter and set aside but within arm's reach.
18. Take the eggs, sweetener, lemon juice, and lemon zest and add it to the top pot. Continue to whisk until the liquids are well combined and thickening.
19. Note: It will thicken suddenly.
20. Once it thickens, take it off of the heat and add in the butter.
21. Continue to whisk until smooth and creamy.
22. Set aside in a glass jar to cool. Put in the fridge until needed.
23. Directions for the Chaffles:
24. Follow the steps for the Classic Sweet Chaffle Recipe.
25. Lay out chaffles individually and spread the lemon curd onto each one followed by one meringue.

26. Enjoy!

201.Brownie Chaffles

Preparation Time: 30 minutes
Cooking Time: 10 minutes
Serving: 1 large chaffles or 2 mini chaffles

Ingredients:

- Classic Sweet Chaffle Recipe

- 1/4 of a cup of dark chocolate cocoa powder

- 1/2 of a cup of Lily's chocolate chips

- 2 tbsp of heavy whipping cream

- 1 tsp of vanilla

- Vanilla Sauce Recipe

- Tools: one mixing bowl, measuring cups and tablespoons, spatula, non-stick cooking spray (or butter), blender, electric beaters, or whisk.

Directions:

1. Follow the steps for the Vanilla Sauce Recipe and put aside.

2. Take a bowl and mix the heavy whipping cream and vanilla until it thickens.

3. Leave in the fridge until ready to serve.

4. Mix the cocoa powder and chocolate chips into the Classic Sweet Chaffle Recipe.

5. Follow the instructions for the Classic Sweet Chaffle Recipe

6. Once ready, lay out two chaffles and spread the whipped cream onto each one and sandwich together. Sprinkle more chocolate chips on top.

7. Enjoy!

202.Tiramisu Chaffle Cake

Preparation Time: 30 minutes
Cooking Time: 10 minutes
Serving: 1 large chaffles or 2 mini chaffles

Chaffle Ingredients:

- Classic Sweet Chaffle Recipe

- Coffee Drizzle Ingredients

- 2 tbsp of very strong coffee

- 1 tsp of brandy extract

- Cream Layer Ingredients

- 4 tbsp of heavy whipping cream

- 4 tbsp of granulated sweetener of choice

- 1 tsp of brandy essence

- Chocolate Drizzle Topping

- three squares of 80-100% chocolate

- Tools: one mixing bowl, measuring cups and tablespoons, spatula, non-stick cooking spray (or butter), blender, electric beaters, or whisk.

Directions:

1. Make a pot of coffee and set aside two tablespoons (feel free to drink the rest!)

2. Mix the coffee and brandy extract together. Set aside.

3. Whip the cream with the sweetener and vanilla extract until thick. Mix in the brandy extract.

4. Leave the whipped cream in the fridge until needed.

5. Follow the instructions for the Sweet Chaffle Recipe.

6. Lay out three chaffles and drizzle the coffee sauce on each one, followed by a dollop of the cream on each one and then sandwich together.

7. Layer the whipped cream on the top of the stack.

8. Take the chocolate and melt it in the

microwave for 15 seconds at a time. Stir after each timed section until fully melted.

9. Drizzle the chocolate on top of the stack.

10. Enjoy!

203.Maple Chaffles

Preparation Time: 30 minutes
Cooking Time: 10 minutes
Serving: 1 large chaffles or 2 mini chaffles

Ingredients:

- Classic Sweet Chaffle Recipe
- 1 tsp of maple extract
- Keto-friendly pancake syrup

Directions:

1. Follow the instructions for the Sweet Chaffle Recipe with the maple extract mixed into the batter.

2. Drizzle the keto-friendly pancake syrup on top of the stack.

3. Enjoy!

204.Cannoli Chaffle

Preparation Time: 30 minutes
Cooking Time: 10 minutes
Serving Size: 1 large chaffles or 2 mini chaffles

Chaffle Ingredients:

- Classic Sweet Chaffle Recipe
- Cannoli Filling Ingredients:
- 2 ounces of cream cheese
- 2 tbsp of confectioner's sweetener, low carb
- 6 tablespoons of ricotta, full fat
- 1/2 teaspoon vanilla extract
- 5 drops of lemon extract

- Lily's Chocolate Chips
- Tools: one mixing bowl, measuring cups and tablespoons, spatula, non-stick cooking spray (or butter), wide bowl, piping bag, blender, electric beaters, or whisk.

Directions:

1. Take all of the cannoli filling and mix together in a bowl until well incorporated.

2. Put the filling into a piping bag and leave in the fridge until ready.

3. Follow instructions for the Sweet Chaffle Recipe.

4. Take a warm chaffle and roll it into a taco shape.

5. Take the piping bag filled with the Cannoli Filling and pipe it into the center of the chaffle until full.

6. Sprinkle a few chocolate chips onto the ends of the cannoli chaffle.

7. Enjoy!

205.Keto Churro Chaffle

Preparation time: 10 minutes
Cooking time: 5 minutes

Ingredients

- 1 egg
- 1/2 cup mozzarella cheese shredded
- 2 tbsp Swerve/ monkfruit Sweetener
- 1/2 teaspoon cinnamon

Directions:

1. Preheat your mini waffle maker.

2. In a small bowl, whip the egg with a fork.

3. Add the shredded cheese to the egg mixture, and mix lightly.

4. Place half of the egg mixture in the

waffle maker and cook it until it's golden brown (for about 3-4 minutes)

5. While the chaffle is cooking, add the sweetener of choice and cinnamon in a separate small bowl.

6. Once the Chaffle is done, cut it into slices while it's still hot and add it to the cinnamon mixture. It soaks up more of the mixture when it's still hot!

7. Serve warm and enjoy.

206.Choco Chip Chaffle

Preparation time: 10 minutes
Cooking time: 5 minutes

Ingredients

- 1 large egg
- 1 teaspoon coconut flour
- 1 teaspoon monkfruit sweetener
- 1/2 teaspoon vanilla extract
- 1/2 cup finely
- shredded mozzarella
- 2 tablespoons sugar-free chocolate chips

Directions:

1. Preheat your waffle maker..

2. Add the egg, coconut flour, sweetener, and vanilla to a small bowl and whisk together with a fork.

3. Stir in the shredded cheese.

4. Spoon half of the batter into the waffle iron and dot with half of the chocolate chips. Spread a bit of batter over each chocolate chip.

5. Close the waffle iron and cook for 3-4 minutes or until as crisp as you'd like.

6. Repeat with remaining batter.

7. Serve hot with whipped cream or low carb ice cream.

207.Vanilla Twinkie Chaffle

Preparation time: 10 minutes
Cooking time: 5 minutes
Servings: 4

Ingredients

- 2 large eggs
- 2 tablespoons butter, melted (cooled)
- 2 ounces cream cheese, softened
- 1 teaspoon vanilla extract
- 1/4 cup almond flour
- 1 teaspoon baking powder
- 2 tablespoons coconut flour
- 1/4 cup Lakanto Confectioners
- Pinch of pink salt
- 1/2 teaspoon Vanilla Cupcake extract (optional)

Directions:

1. Preheat the corndog Maker.

2. Melt the butter and let it cool a minute.

3. Whisk the eggs into the butter until creamy.

4. Add vanilla, extract, and sweetener, salt and then blend well.

5. Add Almond flour, coconut flour, and baking powder and blend until well incorporated.

6. Add ~2 tbs batter to each well and spread across evenly.

7. Cook for 4 minutes.

8. Remove, let it cool, and enjoy.

208.Savory Herb Chaffle

Preparation time: 10 minutes
Cooking time: 5 minutes

Ingredients

- 1 large egg
- 1/4 cup Mozzarella
- 1/4 cup parmesan
- 1/2 Tbsp butter melted
- 1 tsp herb blend seasoning
- 1/2 tsp salt

Directions:

1. Heat your mini waffle maker

2. Holding back a small amount of Mozzarella, mix everything together making sure egg is well incorporated.

3. Put a small amount of Mozzarella onto the bottom of the waffle maker, pour 1/4 mixture on top if the cheese then put more Mozzarella on top.

4. Cook for 4-5 minutes.

5. Let it cool and then enjoy your savory herb chaffle

209.Mint Chocolate Brownie Chaffles

Preparation time: 5 minutes
Cooking time: 5 minutes
Servings: 1

Ingredients:

- 1 cup mint chocolate
- ½ tsp baking powder
- 1 tbsp. cocoa powder
- ½ cup heavy cream
- Sweetener
- 1 cup coconut flour
- ½ tbsp. vanilla extract
- 1 tbsp. butter
- Mint chocolate chips
- 1 egg

Directions:

1. Preheat the waffle maker. In a bowl add coconut flour, egg, baking powder, vanilla extract, cocoa powder and mix them well. In a small bowl add butter and mint chocolate and melt. Pour the melted butter mixture over the ingredients and well combined. Now pour the batter over the waffle maker and cook for 4 to 5 minutes. Repeat the process for all batter. In a separate bowl mix heavy crème with sweetener and vanilla extract until fluffy. Pour the frosting over the chaffles and sprinkle mint chocolate chips. Serve the keto mint chocolate chaffles.

210.Apple Pie Churro Chaffles

Preparation time: 20 minutes
Cooking time: 25 minutes
Servings: 4

Ingredients:

- Apple pie filling:
- 1 tbsp. butter
- 1/8 tsp cream
- 2 tsp cinnamon
- 1/8 tsp nutmeg

Chaffle:

- 2 eggs
- 1 tsp cinnamon
- 2 tsp coconut flour
- 1 tsp vanilla extract
- 2 packet lemon
- ¼ cup swerve
- 1/8 tsp ginger powder
- 1 chayote squash
- ¼ cup mozzarella cheese

- 1 tbsp. swerve
- 1/8 tsp baking powder

Directions:

1. For apple pie filling, mix the butter, lemon, cream, swerve, ginger powder, cinnamon, nutmeg together and coat the chayote with the mixture. After this set into the baking try and cook for 20 minutes. ¼ part of the mixture blend into the mixture to make a sauce. Cook the sauce over medium flame until require consistency achieved. After that stir the chayote into the sauce. For the chaffles, take a bowl and whisk eggs, sweetener, cinnamon, coconut flour, vanilla extract, baking powder, mozzarella cheese and mix until well combined. Pour the batter over the waffle maker and cook until golden brown for 5 minutes. Now place the chaffle in tacos holder and fill it with the apple filling, top it up with cream or vanilla ice cream and serve.

211.Cream Cheese Carrot Chaffles

Preparation time: 10 minutes
Cooking time: 10 minutes
Servings: 1

Ingredients:

- ½ cup carrot
- 2 tbsp. butter
- ¾ cup almond flour
- 2 tbsp. sweetener
- 1 tsp pumpkin sauce
- 4 oz. cream cheese
- 1 tsp vanilla extract
- 1 egg
- 1 tbsp. heavy cream
- 1 tbsp. walnuts

- 2 tsp cinnamon
- 1 tsp. baking powder
- ¼ cup sweetener
- 1-2 tbsp. heavy cream

Directions:

1. In a bowl add almond flour, cinnamon, pumpkin sauce, baking powder, sweetener and walnut and mix. Now add carrot, egg, butter, heavy cream and fold the mixture until well combined. Preheat the waffle maker and pour the batter on the maker. Cook it for 3 minutes. Repeat the procedure for rest of the batter. For frosting pour the cream cheese, sweetener, heavy cream and vanilla extract in a mixture and mix until fluffy. Fill each chaffle with the frosting layer and serve the cream cheese chaffles.

212Keto Mini Cream Cheese Waffles

Preparation time: 3 minutes
Cooking time: 8 minutes
Servings: 2

Ingredients:

- 2 tsp coconut flour
- ¼ tsp baking powder
- 1 oz. cream cheese
- 4 tsp swerve
- 1 egg
- ½ vanilla extract

Directions:

1. Preheat mini waffle maker. Take a bowl whisk egg, crème cheese and vanilla extract until well combined. Now add coconut flour, baking powder, swerve and fold with the batter until smooth. Pour the batter

over the waffle maker and cook for 3 to 4 minutes. Top up the chaffle with the crème cheese and topping of your choice.

213.Keto Double Chocolate Chaffles

Preparation time: 5 minutes
Cooking time: 5 minutes
Servings: 1

Ingredients:

- 1 egg
- 1 oz. cream cheese
- 1 cup dark unsweetened chocolate
- ½ tbsp. cocoa powder
- 1 tbsp. butter
- 1tsp vanilla extract
- 1 tbsp. chocolate syrup
- 1tbsp sweetener
- ¼ tsp baking powder
- 1 cup Coconut flour

Directions:

1. Preheat the waffle maker. In a bowl add coconut flour, baking powder, vanilla extract, egg, chocolate syrup, sweetener and mix them well until well combined. In a separate bowl add butter and a portion of dark chocolate and melt in microwave. Add the chocolate into mixture and fold well. Pour the batter over heated waffle maker and cook for 4 to 5 minutes. Repeat the process for whole batter. Before serving add heavy cream frosting and dark chocolate and enjoy keto double chocolate chaffles.

214.Strawberry & Cream Keto Chaffle

Preparation time: 2 minutes

Cooking time: 5 minutes
Servings: 2

Ingredients:

- 1 egg
- 1 tsp coconut flour
- ½ tsp cake batter extract
- Strawberries
- 1 tbsp. heavy cream
- 2 tbsp. sweetener
- ¼ tsp baking powder

Directions:

1. Preheat waffle maker. In a bowl add coconut flour, egg, cake batter extract, baking powder, sweetener and mix all ingredients well. Pour the mixture over the waffle maker and cook for 4 minutes. Repeat the process for whole batter and prepare chaffles. Add the whipped crème over the chaffles and top up with the strawberries. Serve the keto strawberry crème chaffle.

215.Creamy Chaffle

Preparation time: 5 minutes
Cooking time: 5 minutes
Servings: 2

Ingredients:

- 1 egg, whisked
- 2 tablespoons stevia
- 1 tablespoon heavy cream
- ½ teaspoon almond extract
- 1 teaspoon almond flour
- ½ teaspoon baking soda

Directions:

1. In a bowl, mix the egg with the cream, stevia and the other ingredients and whisk well.

114

2. Preheat the waffle iron at medium-high, pour half of the batter, close the iron, cook the chaffle for 4 minutes and transfer to a plate.

3. Repeat with the rest of the batter and serve warm.

216. Blackberry Chaffle

Preparation time: 5 minutes
Cooking time: 8 minutes
Servings: 4

Ingredients:

- ¼ cup cream cheese, soft
- ¼ cup blackberries
- 2 tablespoons almond flour
- 1 egg, whisked
- 1 tablespoon stevia
- ½ teaspoon baking soda

Directions:

1. In a bowl, mix the cream cheese with the berries and the other ingredients and whisk well.

2. Heat up the waffle iron over high heat, pour ¼ of the batter, close the waffle maker, cook for 8 minutes and transfer to a plate.

3. Repeat with the rest of the batter and serve the chaffles warm.

217. Coconut Chaffle

Preparation time: 5 minutes
Cooking time: 10 minutes
Servings: 4

Ingredients:

- ½ cup cream cheese, soft
- 1 tablespoon coconut flesh, unsweetened and shredded
- 2 teaspoons coconut oil, melted

- 1 tablespoon coconut flour
- 3 eggs, whisked
- 1 tablespoon erythritol
- 1 teaspoon vanilla extract
- ½ teaspoon almond extract

Directions:

1. In a bowl, combine the cream cheese with the melted coconut oil and the other ingredients and whisk well.

2. Heat up the waffle iron over high heat, pour ¼ of the batter, close the waffle maker, cook for 10 minutes and transfer to a plate.

3. Repeat with the rest of the batter and serve the chaffles warm.

218. Vanilla Raspberry Chaffle

Preparation time: 5 minutes
Cooking time: 8 minutes
Servings: 2

Ingredients:

- ½ cup cream cheese, soft
- 1 teaspoon vanilla extract
- 1 tablespoon almond flour
- ¼ cup raspberries, pureed
- 1 egg, whisked
- 1 tablespoon monk fruit

Directions:

1. In a bowl, mix the cream cheese with the raspberry puree and the other ingredients and whisk well.

2. Heat up the waffle iron over high heat, pour half of the batter, close the waffle maker, cook for 8 minutes and transfer to a plate.

3. Repeat with the rest of the batter and serve the chaffles warm.

219.Nutmeg Chaffle

Preparation time: 5 minutes
Cooking time: 5 minutes
Servings: 2

Ingredients:

- 3 tablespoons heavy cream
- 1 tablespoon coconut oil, melted
- 1 tablespoon coconut flour
- 1 egg, whisked
- 1 tablespoon stevia
- ½ teaspoon nutmeg, ground
- 2 tablespoons cream cheese
- ½ teaspoon vanilla extract

Directions:

1. In a bowl, mix the cream with the coconut oil, egg and the other ingredients and whisk well.
2. Heat up the waffle iron over high heat, pour half of the batter, close the waffle maker, cook for 5 minutes and transfer to a plate.
3. Repeat with the remaining batter and serve.

220.Almond Plums Chaffle

Preparation time: 5 minutes
Cooking time: 6 minutes
Servings: 4

Ingredients:

- ½ cup heavy cream
- ½ cup almonds, chopped
- 2 plums, pitted and chopped
- 1 tablespoon almond flour
- 3 eggs, whisked
- 2 tablespoons erythritol
- 1 tbsp. heavy cream

- 2 tbsp. sweetener
- ¼ tsp baking powder
- 2 tablespoons cream cheese

Directions:

1. In a bowl, mix the cream with the almonds, plums and the other ingredients and whisk well.
2. Heat up the waffle iron over high heat, pour ¼ of the batter, close the waffle maker, cook for 6 minutes and transfer to a plate.
3. Repeat with the remaining batter and serve the chaffles warm.

221.Almond Butter Chaffle

Preparation time: 5 minutes
Cooking time: 6 minutes
Servings: 4

Ingredients:

- 4 eggs, whisked
- cup almond flour
- tablespoons swerve
- ½ cup almond butter, soft
- 1 teaspoon baking soda
- teaspoons vanilla extract
- 2 tablespoons coconut oil, melted

Directions:

1. In a bowl, combine the eggs with the almond flour, swerve and the other ingredients and whisk well.
2. Heat up the waffle iron over high heat, pour ¼ of the batter, close the waffle maker, cook for 6 minutes and transfer to a plate.
3. Repeat with the rest batter and serve the chaffles warm.

222.Mint Chaffle

Preparation time: 5 minutes
Cooking time: 5 minutes
Servings: 2

Ingredients:

- ½ cup cream cheese, soft
- tablespoon almond flour
- ½ tablespoon coconut flour
- eggs whisked
- 1 tablespoon swerve
- tablespoons mint, chopped
- 1 teaspoon vanilla extract
- ½ teaspoon almond extract

Directions:

1. In a bowl, combine the cream cheese with the flour and the other ingredients and whisk well.
2. Heat up the waffle iron over high heat, pour half of the batter, close the waffle maker, cook for 5 minutes and transfer to a plate.
3. Repeat with the other part of the batter and serve the chaffles warm.

223.Melon Puree Chaffle

Preparation time: 5 minutes
Cooking time: 5 minutes
Servings: 2

Ingredients:

- ½ cup melon, peeled and pureed
- 3 tablespoons cream cheese, soft
- tablespoon coconut flour
- 1 egg, whisked
- 1 tablespoon stevia
- ½ teaspoon almond extract

Directions:

1. In a bowl, mix the melon puree with the cream cheese and the other ingredients and whisk well.
2. Heat up the waffle iron over high heat, pour half of the batter, close the waffle maker, cook for 5 minutes and transfer to a plate.
3. Repeat with the other part of the batter and serve.

224Sweet Zucchini Chaffle

Preparation time: 5 minutes
Cooking time: 7 minutes
Servings: 4

Ingredients:

- ½ cup zucchinis, grated
- 4 tablespoons cream cheese, soft
- tablespoon almond flour
- 1 tablespoon almonds, chopped
- eggs, whisked
- 1 tablespoon swerve
- ½ teaspoon vanilla extract

Directions:

1. In a bowl, mix the zucchinis with the cream cheese, almond flour and other ingredients and whisk well.
2. Heat up the waffle iron over high heat, pour ¼ of the batter, close the waffle maker, cook for 7 minutes and transfer to a plate.
3. Repeat with the remaining batter and serve the chaffles hot.

225.Pumpkin and Avocado Chaffle

Preparation time: 5 minutes
Cooking time: 5 minutes
Servings: 4

Ingredients:

- ½ cup heavy cream
- avocado, peeled, pitted and mashed
- 1 tablespoon coconut flour
- eggs, whisked
- tablespoons swerve
- 2 and ½ tablespoons pumpkin puree
- 2 tablespoons cream cheese, soft

Directions:

1. In a bowl, combine the cream with the avocado, pumpkin puree and the other ingredients and whisk.
2. Heat up the waffle iron over high heat, pour ¼ of the batter, close the waffle maker, cook for 5 minutes and transfer to a plate.
3. Repeat with the rest of the batter and serve the chaffles warm.

226.Nuts Chaffle

Preparation time: 5 minutes
Cooking time: 8 minutes
Servings: 4

Ingredients:

- 2 tablespoons almonds, chopped
- 2 tablespoons walnuts, chopped
- tablespoon stevia
- ½ cup cream cheese, soft
- eggs, whisked
- 1 tablespoon almond flour
- 1 tablespoon coconut flour
- ½ teaspoon almond extract

Directions:

1. In a blender, mix the almonds with the walnuts, cream cheese and the other ingredients and pulse well.

2. Heat up the waffle iron over high heat, pour ¼ of the batter, close the waffle maker, cook for 5 minutes and transfer to a plate.

3. Repeat with the other part of the batter and serve.

227.Blueberries and Almonds Chaffles

Preparation time: 5 minutes
Cooking time: 8 minutes
Servings: 6

Ingredients:

½ cup cream cheese, soft

- ½ cup blueberries pureed
- 2 tablespoons almonds
- tablespoon almond flour
- eggs, whisked
- 1 and ½ tablespoon stevia
- ½ teaspoon almond extract

Directions:

1. In a bowl, mix the cream cheese with the blueberries, eggs and the other ingredients and whisk well.

2. Heat up the waffle iron over high heat, pour 1/6 of the batter, close the waffle maker, cook for 5 minutes and transfer to a plate.

3. Repeat with the other part of the batter and serve.

228.Rhubarb Chaffles

Preparation time: 5 minutes
Cooking time: 6 minutes
Servings: 3

Ingredients:

- ½ cup rhubarb, chopped
- ¼ cup heavy cream

- 3 tablespoons cream cheese, soft
- 2 tablespoons almond flour
- 2 eggs, whisked
- 2 tablespoons swerve
- ½ teaspoon vanilla extract
- ½ teaspoon nutmeg, ground

Directions:

1. In a bowl, mix the rhubarb with the cream, cream cheese and the other ingredients and whisk well.

2. Heat up the waffle iron over high heat, pour 1/3 of the batter, close the waffle maker, cook for 5 minutes and transfer to a plate.

3. Repeat with the rest of the chaffle batter and serve.

229.Sweet Turmeric Chaffles

Preparation time: 5 minutes
Cooking time: 6 minutes
Servings: 2

Ingredients:

- 3 tablespoons cream cheese, soft
- ½ teaspoon turmeric powder
- ½ teaspoon vanilla extract
- 2 tablespoons coconut flour
- 2 eggs, whisked
- 2 tablespoons stevia

Directions:

1. In a bowl, mix the cream cheese with the turmeric, vanilla and the other ingredients and whisk well.

2. Heat up the waffle iron over high heat, pour ½ of the batter, close the waffle maker, cook for 6 minutes and transfer to a plate.

3. Repeat with the other part of the batter and serve right away.

119

SAVORY CHAFFLES

. 230.Grilled Cheese Chaffle

Preparation time: 3 minutes
Cooking time: 8 minutes
Servings: 1

Ingredients:

- 1 egg
- 1/4 teaspoon garlic powder
- 1/2 cup shred cheddar
- 2 american cheese or 1/4 cup shredded cheese
- 1 tablespoon butter

Directions

1. In a small bowl, mix bacon, garlic powder and shredded cheddar cheese.

2. After heating the dash waffle maker, add half the mixture of the scramble. Cook and cook for 4 minutes.

3. Add to the dash mini waffle maker the remainder of the scramble mixture and cook for 4 minutes.

4. Steam the stove pan over moderate heat when both chaffles are finished.

5. Attach 1 spoonful of butter and dissolve. Place one chaffle in the pan once the butter has melted. Place your favorite cheese on top of the chaffle and finish with a second chaffle.

6. Cook the chaffle for 1 minute on the first side, turn it over and cook for another 1-2 minutes on the other side to finish the cheese melting.

7. Cut it from the bread when the cheese melts and eat it!

Nutrition:

Calories: 549kcal

carbohydrates: 3g
protein: 27g
fats: 48g
saturated fats: 28g
cholesterol: 295mg
sodium: 1216mg
potassium: 172mg
sugar: 1g

.231 Baked Potato Chaffle Using Jicama

Preparation time: 20 minutes
Cooking time: 7 minutes
Servings: 1

Ingredients:

- 1 jicama root
- 1/2 onion, medium, minced
- 2 cloves garlic, pressed
- 1 cup cheese
- 1 eggs, whisked
- Salt and pepper

Directions:

1. Peel the jicama root and shred it using a food processor.

2. Place the shredded jicama root in a colander to allow the water to drain. Mix in 2 tsp of salt as well.

3. Squeeze out the remaining liquid.

4. Microwave the shredded jicama for 5-8 minutes. This step pre-cooks it.

5. Mix all the remaining Ingredients together with the jicama.

6. Start preheating the waffle maker.

7. Once preheated, sprinkle a bit of cheese on the waffle maker, allowing it to toast for a few seconds.

8. Place 3 tbsp of the jicama mixture onto the waffle maker. Sprinkle more cheese on top before closing the lid.

9. Cook for 5 minutes. Flip the chaffle and let it cook for 2 more minutes.

10. Servings your baked jicama by topping it with sour cream, cheese, bacon pieces, and chives.

Nutrition:

calories: 168
carbohydrates: 5.1g
fat: 11.8g
protein: 10g

231 231. . Tiramisu Chaffle

Preparation time: 6 hrs
Cooking time: 6 mins
Servings: 8

Ingredients:

- 2 eggs
- 2 oz cream cheese, softened
- 1 tbsp coconut flour
- 1 tbsp heavy cream
- 1 tsp vanilla extract
- 1/2 tsp baking powder
- 1/2 tsp ground cinnamon
- 1/4 tsp stevia powder
- For the coffee syrup:
- 4 tbsp strong coffee
- 5 drops liquid stevia
- For the filling:
- 1 oz cream cheese, softened
- 3 oz mascarpone cheese, softened
- 1/4 cup heavy cream
- 2 tsp vanilla extract
- 1/4 tsp stevia powder
- For dusting:
- 1/2 tsp unsweetened cocoa powder

Directions:

1. Preheat the mini waffle maker.

2. Combine all the chaffle Ingredients in a blender.

3. Once the waffle maker is heated, pour about 1/4 of the batter and allow it to cook for 5-6 minutes. Remove the cooked chaffle and repeat this step for the remaining batter.

4. While waiting for the chaffle to cook, mix the liquid stevia and coffee in a small bowl for the coffee syrup.

5. For the filling, mix the vanilla, stevia powder, and heavy cream. Whisk this until soft peaks start to form.

6. In a separate mixing bowl, use a hand mixer to combine the mascarpone and cream cheese. Once done, mix it in with the whipped cream.

7. To assemble, drizzle 1 tbsp of coffee syrup on the chaffle.

8. On one chaffle, spread a quarter of the filling. Top this with another chaffle, and repeat the previous step until you have four layers of chaffles.

9. Dust the finished tiramisu chaffle with the unsweetened cocoa powder.

10. Refrigerate this for 6 hours or more before serving.

Nutrition:

calories: 567
carbohydrate: 6.6g
fat: 53.4g
protein: 14.7g

. 232Spicy Jalapeno Popper Chaffles

Preparation time: 10 mins
Cooking time: 10 mins
Servings: 1

Ingredients: for the chaffles:

- 1 egg
- 1 oz cream cheese, softened
- 1 cup cheddar cheese, shredded
- For the toppings:
- 2 tbsp bacon bits
- 1/2 tbsp jalapenos

Directions:

1. Turn on the waffle maker. Preheat for up to 5 minutes.
2. Mix the chaffle Ingredients.
3. Pour the batter onto the waffle maker.
4. Cook the batter for 3-4 minutes until it's brown and crispy.
5. Remove the chaffle and repeat steps until all remaining batter have been used up.
6. Sprinkle bacon bits and a few jalapeno slices as toppings.

Nutrition:

calories: 231
carbohydrate: 2g
fat: 18g
protein: 13g

233. Breakfast Chaffle Sandwich

Preparation time: 15 minutes
Cooking time: 12 minutes
Servings: 1

Ingredients:

- 1 egg
- 1/2 cup monterey jack cheese
- 1 tbsp almond flour
- 2 tbsp butter

Directions:

1. Preheat the waffle maker for 5 minutes until it's hot.

2. Combine monterey jack cheese, almond flour, and the egg in a bowl. Mix well.
3. Take 1/2 of the batter and pour it into the preheated waffle maker. Allow to cook for 3-4 minutes.
4. Repeat previous step for the remaining batter.
5. Melt butter on a small pan. Just like you would with french toast, add the chaffles and let each side cook for 2 minutes. To make them crispier, press down on the chaffles while they cook.
6. Remove the chaffles from the pan. Allow to cool for a few minutes. Servings.

Nutrition:

calories: 514
carbohydrates: 2g
fat: 47g
protein: 21g

234. Peanut Butter And Jelly Chaffles

Preparation time: 10 minutes
Cooking time: 4 minutes
Servings: 1

- 1 egg
- 2 slices cheese, thinly sliced
- 1 tsp natural peanut butter
- 1 tsp sugar-free raspberry
- Cooking spray

Directions:

1. Crack and whisk the egg in a small bowl or a measuring cup.
2. Lightly grease the waffle maker with Cooking spray.
3. Preheat the waffle maker.
4. Once it is heated up, place a slice of cheese on the waffle maker and wait

for it to melt.

5. Once melted, pour the egg mixture onto the melted cheese.

6. Once the egg starts cooking, carefully place another slice of cheese on the waffle maker.

7. Close the lid. Cook for 3-4 minutes.

8. Take out the chaffles and place on a plate.

9. Top the chaffles with whipped cream.

10. Drizzle some natural peanut butter and raspberry preServings on top.

Nutrition:

calories: 337
carbohydrates: 3g
fat: 27g
protein: 21g

235. Halloumi Cheese Chaffles

Preparation time: 15 minutes
Cooking time: 6 minutes
Servings: 1

Ingredients:

- 3 oz halloumi cheese
- 2 tbsp pasta sauce

Directions:

1. Make half-inch thick slices of halloumi cheese.

2. With the waffle maker still turned off, place the cheese slices on it.

3. Turn on the waffle maker and let the cheese cook for 3-6 minutes.

4. Remove from the waffle maker and let it cool.

5. Add low-carb pasta or marinara sauce.

Nutrition:

calories: 333
carbohydrates: 2g
fat: 26g
protein: 22g

236. Chaffles Benedict

Preparation time: 15 minutes
Cooking time: 5 minutes
Servings: 4

Ingredients: for the chaffles:

- 12 eggs
- 1 cup cheddar cheese, shredded
- 8 slices bacon
- For the hollandaise sauce:
- 3 egg yolks
- 1 tbsp lemon juice
- 2 pinches kosher salt
- 1/4 tsp dijon mustard or hot sauce, optional
- 1/2 cup butter, salted

Directions:

1. Preheat the waffle maker.

2. Pour water in a pan and place over medium-high heat.

3. Take 4 eggs and beat them in a bowl. The remaining eggs are for poaching.

4. Once the waffle maker is heated up, sprinkle 1 tbsp of cheese and allow it to toast.

5. Take 1 1/2 tbsp of the beaten eggs and place on the toasted cheese.

6. Once the egg starts cooking, add another layer of sprinkled cheese on top.

7. Close the lid. Cook for 2-3 minutes.

8. Remove the cooked chaffle and repeat the steps until you've created 8 chaffles.

9. Fry bacon and set aside for later.

10. Poach the remaining eggs.

11. To make the sauce, combine lemon juice, salt, egg yolks, and dijon mustard or hot sauce in a bowl.

12. In a separate container, melt the butter in the microwave. Let it cool for a few minutes.

13. Pour the melted butter over the egg yolk mixture.

14. Using an immersion blender, pulse the mixture until it becomes yellow and cloudy. Continue pulsing until the consistency becomes creamy and thick.

15. To Servings, place cooked chaffles on a plate.

16. Place a slice of bacon over each chaffle.

17. Top the bacon with poached egg and drizzle with hollandaise sauce.

Nutrition:

calories: 601
carbohydrates: 1g
fat: 51g
protein: 34g

237. Carnivore Chaffle

Preparation time: 15 minutes
Cooking time: 5 minutes
Servings: 1

Ingredients:

- 1 egg
- 1/3 cup mozzarella cheese
- 1/2 cup pork rinds
- Salt

Directions:

1. Preheat the waffle maker.

2. In a small mixing bowl, mix a pinch of salt with the cheese, egg, and pork rinds.

3. Pour the mixture onto the preheated waffle maker. Close the lid and wait for 3-5 minutes while it cooks. You'll know it's cooked once it already has a golden-brown color.

4. Carefully remove it from the waffle maker and Servings.

Nutrition:

calories: 274
carbohydrates: 1g
fat: 20g
protein: 23g

238. Eggnog Chaffles

Preparation time: 15 minutes
Cooking time: 10 minutes
Servings: 1

Ingredients:

- 1 egg, separated
- 1 egg yolk
- 1/2 cup mozzarella cheese Shredded
- 1/2 tsp spiced rum
- 1 tsp vanilla extract
- 1/4 tsp nutmeg, dried
- A dash of cinnamon
- 1 tsp coconut flour
- For the icing:
- 2 tbsp cream cheese
- 1 tbsp powdered sweetener
- 2 tsp rum or rum extract

Directions:

1. Preheat the mini waffle maker.

2. Mix egg yolk in a small bowl until smooth.

3. Add in the sweetener and mix until the powder is completely dissolved.

4. Add the coconut flour, cinnamon, and nutmeg. Mix well.

5. In another bowl, mix rum, egg white, and vanilla. Whisk until well combined.

6. Throw in the yolk mixture with the egg white mixture. You should be able to form a thin batter.

7. Add the mozzarella cheese and combine with the mixture.

8. Separate the batter into two batches. Put 1/2 of the batter into the waffle maker and let it cook for 6 minutes until it's solid.

9. Repeat until you've used up the remaining batter.

10. In a separate bowl, mix all the icing Ingredients.

11. Top the cooked chaffles with the icing, or you can use this as a dip.

Nutrition:

calories: 266
carbohydrates: 2g
fat: 23g
protein: 13g

239. Cheddar Jalapeno Chaffles

Preparation time: 15 minutes
Cooking time: 10 minutes
Servings: 1

Ingredients:

- 1 egg
- 1/2 cup cheddar cheese shredded
- 1 tbsp almond flour
- 1 tbsp jalapenos
- 1 tbsp olive oil

Directions:

1. Preheat the waffle maker.

2. While waiting for the waffle maker to heat up, mix jalapeno, egg, cheese, and almond flour in a small mixing bowl.

3. Lightly grease the waffle maker with olive oil.

4. In the center of the waffle maker, carefully pour the chaffle batter. Spread the mixture evenly toward the edges.

5. Close the waffle maker lid and wait for 3-4 minutes for the mixture to cook. For an even crispier texture, wait for another 1-2 minutes.

01. Remove the chaffle. Let it cool before serving.

Nutrition:

calories: 509
carbohydrates: 5g
fat: 45g
protein: 23g

240. Cauliflower Chaffle

Preparation time: 5 minutes
Cooking time: 5 minutes
Servings: 1

Ingredients:

- 1/2 cup of rice cauliflower
- 1/4 shredded cheddar
- 1 large egg from which half of the yolk has been removed
- 1 tbsp fine almond flour
- Salt and pepper
- Sprinkle extra cheese on the bottom.

Directions

1. spread the mix on a waffle iron and add more cheese.

2. Cook for 8 minutes.

Note: when immersed in ketchup, it tastes like a hash brown. Oh, it cuts the cheese in half nutrition value

Calories 200
16g fat
11g protein
4g total carbs
2g pure carbohydrate
Fiber2g
Sugar 0g

241. Buffalo Hummus Beef Chaffles

Preparation time: 15 minutes
Cooking time: 32 minutes
Servings: 4

Ingredients:

- 2 eggs
- 1 cup + ¼ cup finely grated cheddar cheese, divided
- 2 chopped fresh scallions
- Salt and freshly ground black pepper to taste
- 2 chicken breasts, cooked and diced
- ¼ cup buffalo sauce
- 3 tbsp low-carb hummus
- 2 celery stalks, chopped
- ¼ cup crumbled blue cheese for topping

Directions:

1. Preheat the waffle iron.
2. In a medium bowl, mix the eggs, 1 cup of the cheddar cheese, scallions, salt, and black pepper,
3. Open the iron and add a quarter of the mixture. Close and cook until crispy, 7 minutes.
4. Transfer the chaffle to a plate and make 3 more chaffles in the same manner.
5. Preheat the oven to 400 f and line a baking sheet with parchment paper. Set aside.
6. Cut the chaffles into quarters and arrange on the baking sheet.
7. In a medium bowl, mix the chicken with the buffalo sauce, hummus, and celery.
8. Spoon the chicken mixture onto each quarter of chaffles and top with the remaining cheddar cheese.
9. Place the baking sheet in the oven and bake until the cheese melts, 4 minutes.
10. Remove from the oven and top with the blue cheese.
11. Servings afterward.

Nutrition:

Calories 552
Fats 28.37g carbs 6.97g net carbs 6.07g protein 59.8g

242. Pulled Pork Chaffle Sandwiches

Preparation time: 20 minutes
Cooking time: 28 minutes
Servings: 4

Ingredients:

- 2 eggs, beaten
- 1 cup finely grated cheddar cheese
- ¼ tsp baking powder
- 2 cups cooked and shredded pork
- 1 tbsp sugar-free bbq sauce
- 2 cups shredded coleslaw mix
- 2 tbsp apple cider vinegar
- ½ tsp salt
- ¼ cup ranch dressing

Directions:

1. Preheat the waffle iron.

2. In a medium bowl, mix the eggs, cheddar cheese, and baking powder.

3. Open the iron and add a quarter of the mixture. Close and cook until crispy, 7 minutes.

4. Transfer the chaffle to a plate and make 3 more chaffles in the same manner.

5. Meanwhile, in another medium bowl, mix the pulled pork with the bbq sauce until well combined. Set aside.

6. Also, mix the coleslaw mix, apple cider vinegar, salt, and ranch dressing in another medium bowl.

7. When the chaffles are ready, on two pieces, divide the pork and then top with the ranch coleslaw. Cover with the remaining chaffles and insert mini skewers to secure the sandwiches.

8. Enjoy afterward.

Nutrition:

Calories 374
Fats 23.61g carbs 8.2g net carbs 8.2g protein 28.05g

243. Okonomiyaki Chaffles

Preparation time: 20 minutes
Cooking time: 28 minutes
Servings: 4

Ingredients:

- For the chaffles:
- 2 eggs, beaten
- 1 cup finely grated mozzarella cheese
- ½ tsp baking powder
- ¼ cup shredded radishes
- For the sauce:
- 2 tsp coconut aminos
- 2 tbsp sugar-free ketchup
- 1 tbsp sugar-free maple syrup
- 2 tsp worcestershire sauce
- For the topping:
- 1 tbsp mayonnaise
- 2 tbsp chopped fresh scallions
- 2 tbsp bonito flakes
- 1 tsp dried seaweed powder
- 1 tbsp pickled ginger

Directions:

1. For the chaffles:

2. Preheat the waffle iron.

3. In a medium bowl, mix the eggs, mozzarella cheese, baking powder, and radishes.

4. Open the iron and add a quarter of the mixture. Close and cook until crispy, 7 minutes.

5. Transfer the chaffle to a plate and make a 3 more chaffles in the same manner.

6. For the sauce:

7. Combine the coconut aminos, ketchup, maple syrup, and worcestershire sauce in a medium bowl and mix well.

8. For the topping:

9. In another mixing bowl, mix the mayonnaise, scallions, bonito flakes, seaweed powder, and ginger

10. To Servings:

11. Arrange the chaffles on four different plates and swirl the sauce on top. Spread the topping on the chaffles and Servings afterward.

Nutrition:

Calories 90
Fats 3.32g carbs 2.97g net carbs 2.17g protein 12.09g

244. Keto Reuben Chaffles

Preparation time: 15 minutes
Cooking time: 28 minutes
Servings: 4

Ingredients:

- For the chaffles:
- 2 eggs, beaten
- 1 cup finely grated swiss cheese
- 2 tsp caraway seeds
- 1/8 tsp salt
- ½ tsp baking powder
- For the sauce:
- 2 tbsp sugar-free ketchup
- 3 tbsp mayonnaise
- 1 tbsp dill relish
- 1 tsp hot sauce
- For the filling:
- 6 oz pastrami
- 2 swiss cheese slices
- ¼ cup pickled radishes

Directions:

1. For the chaffles:
2. Preheat the waffle iron.
3. In a medium bowl, mix the eggs, swiss cheese, caraway seeds, salt, and baking powder.
4. Open the iron and add a quarter of the mixture. Close and cook until crispy, 7 minutes.
5. Transfer the chaffle to a plate and make 3 more chaffles in the same manner.

6. For the sauce:
7. In another bowl, mix the ketchup, mayonnaise, dill relish, and hot sauce.
8. To assemble:
9. Divide on two chaffles; the sauce, the pastrami, swiss cheese slices, and pickled radishes.
10. Cover with the other chaffles, divide the sandwich in halves and Servings.

Nutrition:

Calories 316
Fats 21.78g carbs 6.52g net carbs 5.42g protein 23.56g

245. Pumpkin-Cinnamon Churro Sticks

Preparation time: 10 minutes
Cooking time: 14 minutes
Servings: 2

Ingredients:

- 3 tbsp coconut flour
- ¼ cup pumpkin puree
- 1 egg, beaten
- ½ cup finely grated mozzarella cheese
- 2 tbsp sugar-free maple syrup + more for serving
- 1 tsp baking powder
- 1 tsp vanilla extract
- ½ tsp pumpkin spice seasoning
- 1/8 tsp salt
- 1 tbsp cinnamon powder

Directions:

1. Preheat the waffle iron.
2. Mix all the Ingredients in a medium bowl until well combined.

3. Open the iron and add half of the mixture. Close and cook until golden brown and crispy, 7 minutes.

4. Remove the chaffle onto a plate and make 1 more with the remaining batter.

5. Cut each chaffle into sticks, drizzle the top with more maple syrup and Servings after.

Nutrition:

Calories 219
Fats 9.72g carbs 8.64g net carbs 4.34g protein 25.27g

246. Low Carb Keto Broccoli Cheese Waffles

Preparation time: 5 minutes
Cooking time: 5 minutes
Servings: 2

Ingredients:

- 1 cup broccoli, processed
- 1 cup shredded cheddar cheese
- 1/3 cup grated parmesan cheese
- 2 eggs, beats

Directions

1. spray the Cooking spray on the waffle iron and preheat.

2. Use a powerful blender or food processor to process the broccoli until rice consistency.

3. Mix all Ingredients in a medium bowl.

4. Add 1/3 of the mixture to the waffle iron and cook for 4-5 minutes until golden.

Nutrition:

Calories 160
Total fat 11.8g 18%
Cholesterol 121mg 40%

Sodium 221.8mg 9%
Total carbohydrate 5.1g 2%
Dietary fiber 1.7g 7%
Sugars 1.2g
Protein 10g 20%
Vitamin a 133.5µg 9%
Vitamin c 7.3mg 12%

247. Bagel Seasoning Chaffles

Preparation time: 10 minutes
Cooking time: 20 minutes
Servings: 4

Ingredients

- 1 large organic egg
- 1 cup mozzarella cheese, shredded
- 1 tablespoon almond flour
- 1 teaspoon organic baking powder
- 2 teaspoons bagel seasoning
- ¼ teaspoon garlic powder
- ¼ teaspoon onion powder

Directions:

1. Preheat a mini waffle iron and then grease it.

2. In a medium bowl, put all ingredients and with a fork, mix until well combined.

3. Place ¼ of the mixture into preheated waffle iron and cook for about 3–4 minutes.

4. Repeat with the remaining mixture.

5. Serve warm.

248. Protein Cheddar Chaffles

Preparation time: 15 minutes
Cooking time: 48 minutes
Servings: 8

Ingredients

- ½ cup golden flax seeds meal

- ½ cup almond flour
- 2 tablespoons unflavored whey protein powder
- 1 teaspoon organic baking powder
- Salt and ground black pepper, to taste
- ¾ cup cheddar cheese, shredded
- 1/3 cup unsweetened almond milk
- 2 tablespoons unsalted butter, melted
- 2 large organic eggs, beaten

Directions:

1. Preheat a mini waffle iron and then grease it.
2. In a large bowl, add flax seeds meal, flour, protein powder, and baking powder, and mix well.
3. Stir in the cheddar cheese.
4. In another bowl, add the remaining ingredients and beat until well combined.
5. Add the egg mixture into the bowl with flax seeds meal mixture and mix until well combined.
6. Place desired amount of the mixture into preheated waffle iron.
7. Cook for about 4–6 minutes.
8. Repeat with the remaining mixture.
9. Serve warm.

249. Chicken Jalapeño Chaffles

Preparation time: 10 minutes
Cooking time: 10 minutes
Servings: 2
Ingredients

- ½ cup grass-fed cooked chicken, chopped
- 1 organic egg, beaten

- ¼ cup cheddar cheese, shredded
- 2 tablespoons Parmesan cheese, shredded
- 1 teaspoon cream cheese, softened
- 1 small jalapeño pepper, chopped
- 1/8 teaspoon onion powder
- 1/8 teaspoon garlic powder

Directions:

1. Preheat a mini waffle iron and then grease it.
2. In a medium bowl, put all ingredients and with your hands, mix until well combined.
3. Place half of the mixture into preheated waffle iron and cook for about 4–5 minutes.
4. Repeat with the remaining mixture.
5. Serve warm.

250. Chicken & Bacon Chaffles

Preparation time: 10 minutes
Cooking time: 8 minutes
Servings: 2

Ingredients

- 1 organic egg, beaten
- 1/3 cup grass-fed cooked chicken, chopped
- 1 cooked bacon slice, crumbled
- 1/3 cup pepper jack cheese, shredded
- 1 teaspoon powdered ranch dressing

Directions:

1. Preheat a mini waffle iron and then grease it.
2. In a medium bowl, put all ingredients and with a fork, mix until well combined.

3. Place half of the mixture into preheated waffle iron and cook for about 3–4 minutes or until golden-brown.

4. Repeat with the remaining mixture.

01. Serve warm.

251. Sausage Chaffles

Preparation time: 15 minutes
Cooking time: 1 hour
Servings: 12

Ingredients

- 1 pound gluten-free bulk Italian sausage, crumbled
- 1 organic egg, beaten
- 1 cup sharp cheddar cheese, shredded
- ¼ cup Parmesan cheese, grated
- 1 cup almond flour
- 2 teaspoons organic baking powder

Directions:

1. Preheat a mini waffle iron and then grease it.

2. In a medium bowl, put all ingredients and with your hands, mix until well combined.

3. Place about 3 tablespoons of the mixture into preheated waffle iron and cook for about 3 minutes.

4. Carefully, flip the chaffle and cook for about 2 minutes.

5. Repeat with the remaining mixture.

6. Serve warm.

252. Sausage & Veggie Chaffles

Preparation time: 15 minutes
Cooking time: 20 minutes
Servings: 4

Ingredients

- 1/3 cup unsweetened almond milk
- 4 medium organic eggs
- 2 tablespoons gluten-free breakfast sausage, cut into slices
- 2 tablespoons broccoli florets, chopped
- 2 tablespoons bell peppers, seeded and chopped
- 2 tablespoons mozzarella cheese, shredded

Directions:

1. Preheat a waffle iron and then grease it.

2. In a medium bowl, add the almond milk and eggs and beat well.

3. Place the remaining ingredients and stir to combine well.

4. Place desired amount of the mixture into preheated waffle iron.

5. Cook for about 5 minutes.

6. Repeat with the remaining mixture.

7. Serve warm.

253. Cauliflower & Chives Chaffles

Preparation time: 15 minutes
Cooking time: 1 hour 4 minutes
Servings: 8

Ingredients

- 1½ cups cauliflower, grated
- ½ cup cheddar cheese, shredded
- ½ cup mozzarella cheese, shredded
- ¼ cup Parmesan cheese, shredded
- 3 large organic eggs, beaten
- 3 tablespoons fresh chives, chopped
- ¼ teaspoon red pepper flakes,

crushed

- Salt and ground black pepper, to taste

Directions:

1. Preheat a mini waffle iron and then grease it.

2. In a food processor, place all the ingredients and pulse until well combined.

3. Divide the mixture into 8 portions.

4. Place 1 portion of the mixture into preheated waffle iron and cook for about 8 minutes.

5. Repeat with the remaining mixture.

6. Serve warm.

254. Spinach Chaffles

Preparation time: 15 minutes
Cooking time: 20 minutes
Servings: 4

Ingredients

- 1 large organic egg, beaten
- 1 cup ricotta cheese, crumbled
- ½ cup mozzarella cheese, shredded
- ¼ cup Parmesan cheese, grated
- 4 ounces frozen spinach, thawed and squeezed
- 1 garlic clove, minced
- Salt and ground black pepper, to taste

Directions:

1. Preheat a mini waffle iron and then grease it.

2. In a medium bowl, put all ingredients and with a fork, mix until well combined.

3. Place ¼ of the mixture into preheated waffle iron and cook for about 4–5

minutes.

4. Repeat with the remaining mixture.

5. Serve warm.

255. Zucchini Chaffles

Preparation time: 10 minutes
Cooking time: 10 minutes
Servings: 2

Ingredients

- 1 organic egg, beaten
- ¼ cup mozzarella cheese, shredded
- 2 tablespoons Parmesan cheese, grated
- ½ of small zucchini, grated and squeezed
- ¼ teaspoon dried basil, crushed
- Freshly ground black pepper, to taste

Directions:

1. Preheat a mini waffle iron and then grease it.

2. In a medium bowl, put all ingredients and with a fork, mix until well combined.

3. Place half of the mixture into preheated waffle iron and cook for about 4–5 minutes.

4. Repeat with the remaining mixture.

5. Serve warm.

256. Chicken Chaffles

Preparation time: 10 minutes
Cooking time: 8 minutes
Servings: 2

Ingredients

- 1 1/3 cups grass-fed cooked chicken, chopped

- ½ cup cheddar cheese, shredded
- 1 tablespoon sugar-free BBQ sauce
- 1 organic egg, beaten
- 1 tablespoon almond flour

Directions:

1. Preheat a mini waffle iron and then grease it.
2. In a bowl, put all ingredients and with your hands, mix until well combined.
3. Place half of the mixture into preheated waffle iron and cook for about 4 minutes.
4. Repeat with the remaining mixture.
5. Serve warm.

257. Herb Chaffles

Preparation time: 15 minutes
Cooking time: 12 minutes
Servings: 4

Ingredients

- 4 tablespoons almond flour
- 1 tablespoon coconut flour
- 1 teaspoon mixed dried herbs
- ½ teaspoon organic baking powder
- ¼ teaspoon garlic powder
- ¼ teaspoon onion powder
- Salt and ground black pepper, to taste
- ¼ cup cream cheese, softened
- 3 large organic eggs
- ½ cup cheddar cheese, grated
- 1/3 cup Parmesan cheese, grated

Directions:

1. Preheat a waffle iron and then grease it.

2. In a bowl, mix together the flours, dried herbs, baking powder, and seasoning, and mix well.
3. In a separate bowl, put cream cheese and eggs and beat until well combined.
4. Add the flour mixture, cheddar, and Parmesan cheese, and mix until well combined.
5. Place the desired amount of the mixture into preheated waffle iron and cook for about 2–3 minutes.
6. Repeat with the remaining mixture.
7. Serve warm.

258.. Cauliflower Chaffles

Preparation time: 15 minutes
Cooking time: 32 minutes
Servings: 4

- Ingredients
- 1½ cups cauliflower, grated
- ½ cup cheddar cheese
- ½ cup mozzarella cheese
- ¼ cup Parmesan cheese
- 3 large organic eggs
- 3 tablespoons fresh chives, chopped
- ¼ teaspoon red pepper flakes, crushed
- Salt and ground black pepper, to taste

Directions:

1. Preheat a waffle iron and then grease it.
2. In a food processor, place all the ingredients and pulse until well combined.
3. Place the desired amount of the mixture into preheated waffle iron and cook for about 7–8 minutes.
4. Repeat with the remaining mixture.

5. Serve warm.

259. Jalapeño Chaffles

Preparation time: 5 minutes
Cooking time: 10 minutes
Serving: 2

Ingredients

- 1 organic egg, beaten
- ½ cup cheddar cheese, shredded
- ½ tablespoon jalapeño pepper, chopped

Directions:

1. Preheat a mini waffle iron and then grease it.
2. In a medium bowl, put all ingredients and with a fork, mix until well combined.
3. Place half of the mixture into preheated waffle iron and cook for about 3–5 minutes.
4. Repeat with the remaining mixture.
5. Serve warm.

260. Scallion Chaffles

Preparation time: 10 minutes
Cooking time: 8 minutes
Servings: 2

Ingredients

- 1 organic egg, beaten
- ½ cup mozzarella cheese, shredded
- 1 tablespoon scallion, chopped
- ½ teaspoon Italian seasoning

Directions:

1. Preheat a mini waffle iron and then grease it.
2. In a medium bowl, put all ingredients and with a fork, mix until well combined.

3. Place half of the mixture into preheated waffle iron and cook for about 4 minutes.
4. Repeat with the remaining mixture.
5. Serve warm.

261 Broccoli Chaffles

Preparation time: 10 minutes
Cooking time: 8 minutes
Servings: 2

Ingredients

- 1 organic egg, beaten
- ½ cup cheddar cheese, shredded
- ¼ cup fresh broccoli, chopped
- 1 tablespoon almond flour
- ¼ teaspoon garlic powder

Directions:

1. Preheat a mini waffle iron and then grease it.
2. In a bowl, put all ingredients and mix until well combined.
3. Place half of the mixture into preheated waffle iron and cook for about 4 minutes.
4. Repeat with the remaining mixture.
5. Serve warm.

262. Hot Sauce Jalapeño Chaffles

Preparation time: 10 minutes
Cooking time: 8 minutes
Servings: 2

Ingredients

- ½ cup plus 2 teaspoons cheddar cheese, shredded and divided
- 1 organic egg, beaten
- 6 jalapeño pepper slices

- ¼ teaspoon hot sauce
- Pinch of salt

Directions:

1. Preheat a mini waffle iron and then grease it.
2. In a bowl, add ½ cup of cheese and remaining ingredients and mix until well combined.
3. Place about 1 teaspoon of cheese in the bottom of the waffle maker for about 30 seconds before adding the mixture
4. Place half of the mixture into preheated waffle iron and cook for about 3–4 minutes.
5. Repeat with the remaining cheese and mixture.
6. Serve warm.

263. BBQ Rub Chaffles

Preparation time: 5 minutes
Cooking time: 20 minutes
Servings: 4

Ingredients

- 2 organic eggs, beaten
- 1 cup cheddar cheese, shredded
- ½ teaspoon BBQ rub
- ¼ teaspoon organic baking powder

Directions:

1. Preheat a mini waffle iron and then grease it.
2. In a medium bowl, put all ingredients and with a fork, mix until well combined.
3. Place ¼ of the mixture into preheated waffle iron and cook for about 5 minutes.
4. Repeat with the remaining mixture.

5. Serve warm.

264. Easy Breakfast Chaffle

Preparation time: 10 minutes
Cooking time: 5 minutes
Serving: 2

Ingredients:

- 1 egg, lightly beaten
- 1/2 cup mozzarella cheese, shredded

Directions:

1. Preheat your mini waffle maker.
2. In a bowl, mix egg and shredded cheese until combined.
3. Pour half of the batter in the hot waffle maker and cook until golden brown. Repeat with the remaining batter.
4. Serve and enjoy.

265. Tuna Chaffle

Preparation time: 15 minutes
Cooking time: 10 minutes
Servings: 2

Ingredients:

- 1 egg, lightly beaten
- 1/2 cup cheddar cheese, shredded
  - oz can tuna, drained
- Pinch of salt

Directions:

1. Preheat your waffle maker.
2. In a small bowl, mix egg, cheese, tuna, and salt until combined.
3. Pour half of the batter in the hot waffle maker and cook for 4 minutes or until golden brown. Repeat with the remaining batter.
4. Serve and enjoy.

266. Delicious Garlic Chaffle

Preparation time: 20 minutes
Cooking time: 10 minutes
Servings: 2

Ingredients:

- 1 egg
- 1 tsp coconut flour
- 1 tbsp parmesan cheese, grated
- 1/2 cup cheddar cheese, shredded
- 1/4 tsp baking powder
- 1/2 cup mozzarella cheese, shredded
- 1/4 tsp garlic powder
- 1 tbsp butter, melted
- Pinch of salt

Directions:

1. Preheat the waffle maker.
2. In a small bowl, mix egg, cheddar cheese, parmesan cheese, coconut flour, baking powder, and salt until well combined.
3. Spray waffle maker with cooking spray.
4. Pour half of the batter in the hot waffle maker and cook for 4 minutes or until golden brown. Repeat with the remaining batter.
5. In a small bowl, mix butter and garlic powder.
6. Brush chaffles with butter garlic mixture and top with mozzarella cheese.
7. Broil chaffles until cheese melted.
8. Serve and enjoy.

267. Bacon Chaffle

Preparation time: 20 minutes
Cooking time: 10 minutes
Servings: 6

Ingredients:

- 1 egg, lightly beaten
- 1/2 tsp baking powder, gluten-free
- 1/2 tsp dried parsley
- 1/4 tsp onion powder
- 1/4 tsp garlic powder
- 1/4 tsp Swerve
- 1 cup cheddar cheese, shredded
- 1 1/2 tbsp butter, melted
- 4 bacon slices, cooked and crumbled
- 1/4 cup sour cream
- 1/2 cup almond flour

Directions:

1. Preheat your mini waffle maker.
2. In a bowl, mix almond flour, garlic powder, onion powder, and baking powder until combined.
3. In another bowl, add egg, cheese, butter, bacon, parsley, sour cream, and bacon and mix until combined.
4. Add almond flour mixture into the egg mixture and mix well.
5. Pour 2-3 tablespoons of batter in the hot waffle maker and cook for 5-6 minutes or until golden brown. Repeat with the remaining batter.
6. Serve and enjoy.

268 Savoury Cheddar Cheese Chaffle

Preparation time: 10 minutes
Cooking time: 5 minutes
Servings: 1

Ingredients:

- 1 egg
- 1/4 tsp garlic powder

- 1/4 tsp onion powder
- 1/4 tsp baking powder, gluten-free
- 2 tbsp almond flour
- 1/4 cup cheddar cheese, shredded
- Pinch of salt

Directions:

1. Preheat your waffle maker.
2. In a bowl, whisk together egg, garlic powder, baking powder, onion powder, almond flour, cheese, and salt.
3. Spray waffle maker with cooking spray.
4. Pour batter in the hot waffle maker and cook for 3-5 minutes or until set.
5. Serve and enjoy.

269. Perfect Jalapeno Chaffle

Preparation time: 15 minutes
Cooking time: 10 minutes
Servings: 6

Ingredients:

- 3 eggs
- 1 cup cheddar cheese, shredded
- 8 oz cream cheese
- 2 jalapeno peppers, diced
- 4 bacon slices, cooked and crumbled
- 1/2 tsp baking powder
- 3 tbsp coconut flour
- 1/4 tsp sea salt

Directions:

1. Preheat your waffle maker.
2. In a small bowl, mix coconut flour, baking powder, and salt.
3. In a medium bowl, beat cream cheese

using a hand mixer until fluffy.

4. In a large bowl, beat eggs until fluffy.
5. Add cheddar cheese and half cup cream in eggs and beat until well combined.
6. Add coconut flour mixture to egg mixture and mix until combined.
7. Add jalapeno pepper and stir well.
8. Spray waffle maker with cooking spray.
9. Pour 1/4 cup batter in the hot waffle maker and cook for 4-5 minutes. Repeat with the remaining batter.
10. Once chaffle is slightly cool then top with remaining cream cheese and bacon.
11. Serve and enjoy.

270. Crunchy Zucchini Chaffle

Preparation time: 15 minutes
Cooking time: 10 minutes
Servings: 8

Ingredients:

- 2 eggs, lightly beaten
- 1 garlic clove, minced
- 1 1/2 tbsp onion, minced
- 1 cup cheddar cheese, grated
- 1 small zucchini, grated and squeeze out all liquid

Directions:

1. Preheat your waffle maker.
2. In a bowl, mix eggs, garlic, onion, zucchini, and cheese until well combined.
3. Spray waffle maker with cooking spray.
4. Pour 1/4 cup batter in the hot waffle maker and cook for 5 minutes or until

golden brown. Repeat with the remaining batter.

5. Serve and enjoy.

271. Simple Cheese Bacon Chaffles

Preparation time: 10 minutes
Cooking time: 10 minutes
Servings: 4

Ingredients:

- 2 eggs, lightly beaten
- 1/4 tsp garlic powder
- 2 bacon slices, cooked and chopped
- 3/4 cup cheddar cheese, shredded

Directions:

1. Preheat your mini waffle maker and spray with cooking spray.

2. In a bowl, mix eggs, garlic powder, bacon, and cheese.

3. Pour 2 tbsp of the batter in the hot waffle maker and cook for 2-3 minutes or until set. Repeat with the remaining batter.

4. Serve and enjoy.

272. Cheddar Cauliflower Chaffle

Preparation time: 10 minutes
Cooking time: 5 minutes
Servings: 1

Ingredients:

- 1 egg, lightly beaten
- 1 tbsp almond flour
- 1/4 cup cheddar cheese, shredded
- 1/2 cup cauliflower rice
- Pepper
- Salt

Directions:

1. Preheat your waffle maker.

2. Add all ingredients into the bowl and mix until well combined.

3. Spray waffle maker with cooking spray.

4. Pour batter in the hot waffle maker and cook for 8 minutes or until golden brown.

5. Serve and enjoy.

273. Perfect Keto Chaffle

Preparation time: 10 minutes
Cooking time: 8 minutes
Servings: 2

Ingredients:

- 2 eggs, lightly beaten
- 1/2 cup mozzarella cheese, shredded
- 1/2 cup cheddar cheese, shredded
- 1/4 tsp baking powder, gluten-free
- 1 tbsp almond flour
- 1/4 tsp cinnamon
- 1/4 tsp red chili flakes
- 1/4 tsp salt

Directions:

1. Preheat your waffle maker and spray with cooking spray.

2. In a bowl, whisk eggs with baking powder, almond flour, and salt.

3. Add remaining ingredients and mix until well combined.

4. Pour half of the batter in the hot waffle maker and cook for 3-5 minutes or until golden brown. Repeat with the remaining batter.

5. Serve and enjoy.

274. Cabbage Chaffle

Preparation time: 15 minutes
Cooking time: 5 minutes
Servings: 2

Ingredients:

- 1 egg, lightly beaten
- 1/3 cup mozzarella cheese, grated
- ½ bacon slice, chopped
- 1 ½ tbsp green onion, sliced
- 2 tbsp cabbage, chopped
- 2 tbsp almond flour
- Pepper
- Salt

Directions:

1. Add all ingredients in a bowl and stir to combine.
2. Spray waffle maker with cooking spray.
3. Pour half of the batter in the hot waffle maker and cook until golden brown. Repeat with the remaining batter.
4. Serve and enjoy.

275. Simple Ham Chaffle

Preparation time: 10 minutes
Cooking time: 8 minutes
Servings: 2

Ingredients:

- 1 egg, lightly beaten
- 1/4 cup ham, chopped
- 1/2 cup cheddar cheese, shredded
- 1/4 tsp garlic salt
- For Dip:
- 1 1/2 tsp Dijon mustard
- 1 tbsp mayonnaise

Directions:

1. Preheat your waffle maker.
2. Whisk eggs in a bowl.
3. Stir in ham, cheese, and garlic salt until combine.
4. Spray waffle maker with cooking spray.
5. Pour half of the batter in the hot waffle maker and cook for 3-4 minutes or until golden brown. Repeat with the remaining batter.
6. For Dip: In a small bowl, mix mustard and mayonnaise.
7. Serve chaffle with dip.

276. Delicious Bagel Chaffle

Preparation time: 10 minutes
Cooking time: 8 minutes
Servings: 2

Ingredients:

- 1 egg, lightly beaten
- 1/4 tsp garlic powder
- 1/4 tsp onion powder
- 1 1/2 tsp bagel seasoning
- 3/4 cup mozzarella cheese, shredded
- 1/2 tsp baking powder, gluten-free
- 1 tbsp almond flour

Directions:

1. Preheat your waffle maker.
2. In a bowl, mix egg, bagel seasoning, baking powder, onion powder, garlic powder, and almond flour until well combined.
3. Add cheese and stir well.
4. Spray waffle maker with cooking spray.
5. Pour 1/2 of batter in the hot waffle

maker and cook for 5 minutes or until golden brown. Repeat with the remaining batter.

6. Serve and enjoy.

277. Cheesy Garlic Bread Chaffle

Preparation time: 10 minutes
Cooking time: 8 minutes
Servings: 2

Ingredients:

- 1 egg, lightly beaten
- 1 tsp parsley, minced
- 2 tbsp parmesan cheese, grated
- 1 tbsp butter, melted
- 1/4 tsp garlic powder
- 1/4 tsp baking powder, gluten-free
- 1 tsp coconut flour
- 1/2 cup cheddar cheese, shredded

Directions:

1. Preheat your waffle maker.
2. In a bowl, whisk egg, garlic powder, baking powder, coconut flour, and cheddar cheese until well combined.
3. Spray waffle maker with cooking spray.
4. Pour half of the batter in the hot waffle maker and cook for 3 minutes or until set. Repeat with the remaining batter.
5. Brush chaffles with melted butter.
6. Place chaffles on baking tray and top with parmesan cheese and broil until cheese melted.
7. Garnish with parsley and serve.

278. Zucchini Basil Chaffle

Preparation time: 10 minutes
Cooking time: 8 minutes

Servings: 2

Ingredients:

- 1 egg, lightly beaten
- 1/4 cup fresh basil, chopped
- 1/4 cup mozzarella cheese, shredded
- 1/2 cup parmesan cheese, shredded
- 1 cup zucchini, grated and squeeze out all liquid
- 1/4 tsp pepper
- 3/4 tsp salt

Directions:

1. Preheat your waffle maker.
2. In a small bowl, beat the egg.
3. Add basil, mozzarella cheese, zucchini, pepper, and salt and stir well.
4. Spray waffle maker with cooking spray.
5. Sprinkle 2 tbsp of parmesan cheese to the bottom of waffle iron then spread 1/4 of the batter and top with 2 tbsp parmesan cheese and cook for 4-8 minutes or until set. Repeat with the remaining batter.
6. Serve and enjoy.

279. Jicama Chaffle

Preparation time: 10 minutes
Cooking time: 8 minutes
Servings: 2

Ingredients:

- 2 eggs, lightly beaten
- 1 cup cheddar cheese, shredded
- 1/4 tsp garlic powder
- 1/4 tsp onion powder
- 1 large jicama root, peel, shredded and squeeze out all liquid

- Pepper
- Salt

Directions:

1. Preheat your waffle maker.
2. Add shredded jicama in microwave-safe bowl and microwave for 5-8 minutes.
3. Add remaining ingredients to the bowl and stir to combine.
4. Spray waffle maker with cooking spray.
5. Pour half of the batter in the hot waffle maker and cook until golden brown or set. Repeat with the remaining batter.
6. Serve and enjoy.

280. Bacon & Chicken Ranch Chaffle

Preparation Time: 5 minutes
Cooking Time: 8 minutes
Servings: 2

Ingredients:

- 1 egg
- ¼ cup chicken cubes, cooked
- 1 slice bacon, cooked and chopped
- ¼ cup cheddar cheese, shredded
- 1 teaspoon ranch dressing powder

Directions:

1. Preheat your waffle maker.
2. In a bowl, mix all the ingredients.
3. Add half of the mixture to your waffle maker.
4. Cover and cook for 4 minutes.
5. Make the second chaffle using the same steps.

281. Pumpkin & Pecan Chaffle

Preparation Time: 5 minutes
Cooking Time: 10 minutes
Servings: 2
Ingredients:

- 1 egg, beaten
- ½ cup mozzarella cheese, grated
- ½ teaspoon pumpkin spice
- 1 tablespoon pureed pumpkin
- 2 tablespoons almond flour
- 1 teaspoon sweetener
- 2 tablespoons pecans, chopped

Directions:

1. Turn on the waffle maker.
2. Beat the egg in a bowl.
3. Stir in the rest of the ingredients.
4. Pour half of the mixture into the device.
5. Seal the lid.
6. Cook for 5 minutes.
7. Remove the chaffle carefully.
8. Repeat the steps to make the second chaffle.

282. Cheeseburger Chaffle

Preparation Time: 15 minutes
Cooking Time: 15 minutes
Servings: 2

Ingredients:

- 1 lb. ground beef
- 1 onion, minced
- 1 tsp. parsley, chopped
- 1 egg, beaten
- Salt and pepper to taste
- 1 tablespoon olive oil

- 4 basic chaffles
- 2 lettuce leaves
- 2 cheese slices
- 1 tablespoon dill pickles
- Ketchup
- Mayonnaise

Directions:

1. In a large bowl, combine the ground beef, onion, parsley, egg, salt and pepper.
2. Mix well.
3. Form 2 thick patties.
4. Add olive oil to the pan.
5. Place the pan over medium heat.
6. Cook the patty for 3 to 5 minutes per side or until fully cooked.
7. Place the patty on top of each chaffle.
8. Top with lettuce, cheese and pickles.
9. Squirt ketchup and mayo over the patty and veggies.
10. Top with another chaffle.

283. Double Choco Chaffle

Preparation Time: 5 minutes
Cooking Time: 10 minutes
Servings: 2

Ingredients:

- 1 egg
- 2 teaspoons coconut flour
- 2 tablespoons sweetener
- 1 tablespoon cocoa powder
- ¼ teaspoon baking powder
- 1 oz. cream cheese
- ½ teaspoon vanilla
- 1 tablespoon sugar-free chocolate

chips

Directions:

1. Put all the ingredients in a large bowl.
2. Mix well.
3. Pour half of the mixture into the waffle maker.
4. Seal the device.
5. Cook for 4 minutes.
6. Uncover and transfer to a plate to cool.
7. Repeat the procedure to make the second chaffle.

284. Ketogenic Wafers with Almond Flour

Preparation time: 10 minutes
Cooking time: 10 minutes
Servings: 3

Ingredients

- 4 eggs
- 200g cream cheese
- 80g almond flour (e.g. Mea Vita almond flour)
- ½ tsp ground vanilla (e.g. Azafran vanilla powder)
- 1 teaspoon Baking powder

Directions:

1. Mix the eggs and cream cheese in a bowl, and then add the remaining ingredients. Heat a chaffleiron, brush the plates with a little butter and bake 6 chaffles.

285. Ketogenic Wafers with Coconut Flour

Preparation time: 30 minutes
Cooking time: 10 minutes
Servings: 8

Ingredients

- 5 eggs
- 40g coconut flour (e.g. Naturacereal organic coconut flour)
- 1 teaspoon Baking powder
- 3 tbsp unsweetened almond milk (e.g. Alpro unsweetened almond milk)
- 120g butter (e.g. from grass-fed cows)
- 1 tbsp coconut oil (e.g. Mituso organic coconut oil)

Directions:

01. The butter melts and let cool. Separate the eggs and beat the egg whites until stiff. In another bowl, mix egg yolk with coconut flour and baking powder and then slowly stir in the liquid butter.

02. Next add almond milk and vanilla flavor. Finally carefully fold in the egg whites. Heat up a chaffle iron with a little coconut oil grease. Then put the dough for 8 chaffles on the iron and bake.

286. Ketogenic Wafers without Flour

Preparation time: 30 minutes
Cooking time: 10 minutes
Servings: 2

Ingredients

- 2 eggs
- 30g butter
- 50g curd cheese
- ½ tsp psyllium husk (e.g. Vita Natura Indian psyllium husk)
- 3 tbsp protein powder (e.g. ESN whey protein flavor vanilla)
- 1 tbsp coconut oil (e.g. Mituso organic coconut oil)

Directions:

01. The butter melt and let cool. Then stir all the ingredients together thoroughly. A chaffle maker to make hot and the coconut oil grease. Add the dough in portions and even bake. Depending on which protein powder you use, you can make sweet or savory chaffles.

287. Cheese and Bacon Chaffles

Preparation time: 10 minutes
Cooking time: 5 minutes
Servings: 1

Ingredients

- 2 egg
- 30g bacon
- 50g minced meat
- 50g grated cheese (e.g. Emmentaler)
- 1 tsp butter (e.g. from grass-fed cows)

Directions:

1. Cut the bacon into small cubes or strips and fry in a pan until crispy for 1-2 minutes. Mix the egg and cheese thoroughly in a bowl. Finally add the bacon and minced meat to the egg and stir. Heat a chaffle iron and grease it with a little butter so that nothing sticks.

2. Pour the dough onto the chaffle iron and fry until it is as crispy as desired.

288. Raspberry Chaffle

Preparation time: 15 minutes
Cooking time: 5 minutes
Servings: 2

Ingredients

- 60g raspberries (fresh or frozen)
- 1 pinch of cinnamon (e.g. Azafran Bio-

Ceylon cinnamon)

Directions:

1. Simmer the raspberries in a small saucepan until you get a sauce. Then add the cinnamon and pour the raspberry sauce directly and hot over the chaffles.

289. Ketogenic Chaffles

Preparation time: 25 minutes
Cooking time: 10 minutes
Servings: 6

Ingredients

- 75 g almond flour
- 25 g vanilla protein powder
- 2 eggs
- 120 ml almond milk
- 2 tbsp coconut oil
- 1 vanilla bean
- 2 tbsp erythritol
- 1/2 tbsp baking powder

Directions:

1. Mix all the dry ingredients together. Take a knife and cut the vanilla bean, scrape out the pulp with the tip of a knife and add it to the ingredients.

2. Add the eggs just like the melted coconut oil and little by little, stirring the milk.

290. Low Carb Keto Chaffle Recipe Jalapeno Cheddar

Preparation time: 10 minutes
Cooking time: 5 minutes
Servings: 2

Ingredients

- 80 g cream cheese

- 3 eggs
- 1 EL coconut flour
- 1 tsp psyllium seed husks
- 1 tsp baking powder
- 30 g cheddar cheese
- 1 jalapeno
- salt
- pepper

Directions:

1. Put all the ingredients in a bowl.

2. Mix them with a hand blender until the mixture has become an evenly fine chaffle batter.

3. Turn on the chaffle maker.

4. As soon as the chaffle iron is hot enough, pour in the chaffle batter.

5. Take out the low carb chaffle if it has the right consistency for your taste.

6. Now you can serve the chaffle.

291. Chaffles with Raspberry Curd

Preparation time: 30 minutes
Cooking time: 10 minutes
Servings: 2

Ingredients

- For the chaffles:
- 3 eggs (M)
- 75 g cream
- 3 tbsp psyllium husk powder
- salt
- For the curd:
- 50 g raspberries
- 200 g curd cheese (40% fat in dry matter)
- 50 g Greek yogurt

- Moreover:
- Chaffle iron
- Soft butter for greasing

Directions:

1. Mix the eggs, cream, psyllium husk powder, 1 pinch of salt and 150 ml of cold water with the whisk to smooth dough. Let the dough soak for about 5 minutes.

2. In the meantime, select the raspberries, wash carefully and pat dry. Crush something in a bowl with a fork. Add the curd and yogurt and mix everything until creamy.

3. Heat the chaffle iron to a medium setting. Then grease the baking surfaces thinly with the butter using a baking brush. Put a quarter of the dough in the chaffle iron and bake in 3-4 minutes light brown and crispy. Remove and keep warm covered on a plate. Bake three more chaffles from the rest of the dough in the same way. Arrange on two plates and serve with the curd.

292. Sweet Chaffle

Preparation time: 1 minute
Cooking time: 3 minutes
Servings: 1

Ingredients:

- 2 oz cream cheese
- 1 egg
- 1 tablespoon coconut powder
- 2 tsp cocoa
  - cups of sweetener (can be used between 2-3, but 2.5 is preferred)
- 1 teaspoon of vanilla
- 1/2 teaspoon baking soda

- 1 tsp cinnamon (optional)
- Coconut oil spray
- Waffle maker
- 1 teaspoon of butter (optional)

Directions:

2. Place cream cheese for 20 seconds in a microwave safe bowl and microwave. (If your cream cheese is at room temperature, this move is not required.) Combine the rest of your sweet ingredients with the cream cheese in the tub.

3. Plug in your coconut oil waffle maker and spray.

4. Only spoon enough of the combined ingredients of the delicious chaffle on to the waffle maker.

5. Open your waffle maker and wait patiently, yes-it's going to be difficult.

6. Depending on your waffle maker, the exact cooking time varies. We notice that in about 2 minutes most waffle makers cook the delicious chaffles.

7. Take your sweet, cooked chaffle and put it on a plate.

8. Top with a butter slice.

9. Enjoy!

NOTES: If you're not an individual with cinnamon, you should take the ingredient absolutely out of your delicious chaffles. We hope this recipe for keto dessert will be your new favorite! If you like it as much as we do, please share it with your friends on social media.

293. Keto Tuna Melt Chaffle

Preparation time: 5 minutes
Cooking time: 5 minutes
Servings: 2

Ingredients:

- o   oz 1 packet tuna
- 1/2 cup mozzarella cheese
- 1 egg
- Pinch salt

Directions:

1. In a small bowl, preheat the mini waffle maker, add the egg and whip it.

2. Stir in the fish, butter, salt and combine well.

3. Add a teaspoon of cheese to the mini waffle maker for about 30 seconds before adding the mixture of the formula. When the tuna chaffle is cooked, this will allow the cheese to get crispy. This is the form I use!

4. Attach 1/2 of the waffle maker mixture and cook for at least 4 minutes.

5. Cut it and cook another 4 minutes of the last tuna chaffle.

Notes: This recipe produces two chaffles of tuna. If you use a full-size waffle maker, double the recipe.

294. Broccoli & Cheddar Keto Waffles

Preparation time: 5 minutes
Cooking time: 5 minutes
Servings: 1

Ingredients:

- ⅓ Raw broccoli, finely chopped 20 g
- ¼ cup cheddar cheese, shredded 28g
- 1 egg
- 1/2 teaspoon garlic powder
- 1/2 tsp dried onion
- Salt and pepper flavor
- Cooking spray

Directions:

1. To reach the temperature, insert a waffle iron.

2. Beat the egg with a fork in a small bowl.

3. Fold in broccoli, cheese, powdered garlic, onions, salt, pepper.

4. Use cooking spray as soon as the waffle iron is ready (if needed) and add the egg mixture. Cover well waffle iron and apply heat till the light indicates that one cycle is complete.

5. Close the lid again and cook for another period.

6. When finished, gently remove the waffle iron with a tongue or fork.

7. Enjoy! Enjoy! Serve with honey, sour cream, pasture and other sauces.

8. Note: This recipe makes one or two mini waffles at full size.

9. Sprinkle with crushed cheddar cheese before and after spreading the egg mixture.

295. Maple Cream Cheese Icing

Preparation time: 5 minutes
Cooking time: 10 minutes
Servings: 5

Ingredients:

- 4 oz cream cheese
- 1/2 cup heavy cream
- 1/4 cup lacanto maple flavor syrup
- 1 teaspoon of vanilla essence
- 1/4 teaspoon of cinnamon

Directions:

1. Combine softened cream cheese and all other ingredients in a blender

2. Start with a pulse to combine before

blending until smooth

296. Cinnamon Roll Chaffles With Cream Cheese Frosting

Preparation time: 5 minutes
Cooking time: 5 minutes
Servings: 1

Ingredients:

- 1 tbsp cream cheese, tender (or an alternative to sour cream or ricotta cheese)
- One large egg
- 1 teaspoon of melted butter
- 2 tablespoons almond flour (or 1 tablespoon coconut powder)
- 1/4 teaspoon baking powder
- 1 teaspoon ground cinnamon
- 1/2 teaspoon vanilla extract
- 1/4 teaspoon of cinnamon extract (or add 1/2 teaspoon of cinnamon)
- 6-8 drops of LaKanto Monkfruit extract to taste (or 2 teaspoons of granular erythritol)
- Cream cheese frosting ingredients:
- 1 oz cream cheese, softened
- 2 teaspoons powdered erythritol or taste
- 1 teaspoon of vanilla essence
- 1-2 tablespoons of heavy cream

Directions:

1. Preheat a waffle maker with a mini 4. (If you use a regular size waffle maker, double or triple the recipe.) Mix all the ingredients until a smooth batter forms. (If necessary, microwave the cold cream cheese for about 5-8 seconds to soften before adding the remaining ingredients.)

Divide the batter into two and cook each cake for 4 minutes until well browned and crispy. Two mini 4 "chaffles are made from this recipe.

2. Whisk together the whole frosting components in a small bowl and add enough heavy cream to achieve the desired consistency of spreading. Spread the frosting on the warm chaffles and add extra cinnamon to sprinkle. Enjoy! Enjoy!

297. Keto Pumpkin Cheesecake Chaffle

Preparation time: 2 minutes
Cooking time: 4 minutes
Servings: 2

Ingredients:

- Pumpkin chaffle
- 1 egg
- 1/2 cup mozzarella cheese
- 1 1/2 tbsp pumpkin puree (100% pumpkin)
- 1 tablespoon almond flour
- 1 tbsp. Of La Canto Golden Sweetener or Sweetener Choice
- 2 tsp heavy cream
- 1 teaspoon cream cheese
- 1/2 tsp pumpkin spice
- 1/2 teaspoon baking powder
- 1/2 teaspoon vanilla
- 1 teaspoon chocolate zero maple syrup or 1/8 teaspoon maple extract
- Filling
- 2 tablespoons cream cheese
- 1 tablespoon Lakant powder sweetener
- 1/4 teaspoon of vanilla essence

Directions:

1. Preheating mini waffle maker

2. In a small bowl, mix all chaffle ingredients.

3. Pour half of the chaffle mixture into the center of the waffle iron. Cook for 3-5 minutes.

4. Carefully remove and repeat the second chaffle. While making the filling, set it to the crunchy side.

5. With a whisk or fork, mix all the matte ingredients together. Add a frost between the two chaffles. pleasant!

6. Optional: add whipped cream top, crushed pecans, chocolate zero maple syrup and more.

298. Cinnamon Apple Chaffle

Preparation time: 10 minutes
Cooking time: 5 minutes
Servings: 4

Ingredients:

- Vanilla beans sauce:
- 1/2 teaspoon monk fruit sweetener
- 1/2 teaspoon vanilla essence
- 1 egg yolk
- 1 cup whipped cream
- 1 tablespoon ghee or butter
- 2 oz cream cheese softened
- Whole vanilla bean
- Chaffle:
- 2 tablespoons coconut powder
- 1 teaspoon baking powder
- 2 tsp cinnamon
- 1/2 teaspoon monk fruit sweetener
- 3 large eggs
- ¼ cup granny smith apple skin + dice

(or 1 tablespoon of natural erythritol apple flavor)

- ¾chop mozzarella cheese shredded
- ¼chop mild cheddar cheese shredded

Directions:

1. Vanilla Bean Sauce: Add heavy cream, ghee, and vanilla bean to a mild sauce.

2. Heat over medium high heat, then add sweetener and lower heat and cook for 10 minutes. Remove the vanilla bean into whipping cream and scrape the remaining vanilla seeds, then discard the bean.

3. Remove from heat and stir vigorously in egg yolk.

4. Apply cream cheese until the cheese is melted.

5. Put the vanilla sauce in a heat-safe container and cool in the refrigerator.

6. Apple Chaffle: Preheat waffle maker with low carb non-stick spray and spray generously.

7. Add egg and beat in a large mixing bowl until frothy.

8. Add vanilla and cheese and beat until thoroughly combined.

9. Whisk flour, baking powder, sweetener, and cinnamon in a small mixing bowl.

10. To egg mixture, add dry ingredients and mix until combined.

11. Fold gently in the diced apples.

12. Fluid the cooking spray from the waffle maker

13. Pour batter on low, high heat into the waffle maker and cook until the outside starts to brown–about 4 minutes.

14. Slightly cool "hole" and then top with vanilla sauce.

299. Peanut Butter & Jelly Sammich Chaffle

Preparation time: 5 minutes
Cooking time: 5 minutes
Servings: 2

Ingredients:

- Ingredients for chaffle
- 2 eggs
- 1/4 cup mozzarella cheese
- 1 tsp cinnamon
- 1 T confectionery
- Coconut flower 2 tsp
- 1/8 teaspoon baking powder
- 1 teaspoon of vanilla essence
- Blueberry compote ingredients
- 1 cup of washed blueberries
- 1/2 lemon peel
- Freshly squeezed 1 T lemon juice
- 1 T confectionery
- 1/8 teaspoon xanthan gum
- 2 T water

Directions:

1. Add everything except xanthan gum to a small pot.
2. Bring to a boil, lower the heat and cook for 5-10 minutes until it starts to thicken.
3. Sprinkle xanthan gum and stir well.
4. Remove from heat and cool.
5. Keep in refrigerator until ready to use.

300. Pandan Asian Chaffles

Preparation Time: 3 min
Cooking Time: 8 min
Servings: 2

Ingredients

- ½ cup cheddar cheese, finely shredded
- 1 egg
- 3 drops of pandan extract
- 1 tbsp almond flour
- 1/3 tsp garlic powder

Directions:

1. Warm up your mini waffle maker.
2. Mix the egg, almond flour, garlic powder with cheese in a small bowl.
3. Add pandan extract to the cheese mixture and mix well.
4. For a crispy crust, add a teaspoon of shredded cheese to the waffle maker and cook for 30 seconds.
5. Then, pour the mixture into the waffle maker and cook for 5 minutes or until crispy.
6. Repeat with remaining batter.
7. Serve with fried chicken wings with bbq sauce and enjoy!

301. Ham and Jalapenos Chaffle

Preparation Time: 5 min
Cooking Time: 9 min
Servings: 3

Ingredients

- 2 lbs cheddar cheese, finely grated
- 2 large eggs
- ½ jalapeno pepper, finely grated
- 2 ounces ham steak
- 1 medium scallion
- 2 tsp coconut flour

Directions

1. Shred the cheddar cheese using a fine

grater.

2. Deseed the jalapeno and grate using the same grater.

3. Finely chop the scallion and ham.

4. Pour all the ingredients in a medium bowl and mix well.

5. Spray your waffle iron with cooking spray and heat for 3 minutes.

6. Pour 1/4 of the batter mixture into the waffle iron.

7. Cook for 3 minutes, until crispy around the edges.

8. Remove the waffles from the heat and repeat until all the batter is finished.

9. Once done, allow them to cool to room temperature and enjoy.

302. Hot Ham Chaffles

Preparation Time: 5 min
Cooking Time: 4 min
Servings: 2

Ingredients

- ½ cup mozzarella cheese, shredded
- 1 egg
- ¼ cup ham, chopped
- ¼ tsp salt
- 2 tbsp mayonnaise
- 1 tsp Dijon mustard

Directions:

1. Preheat your waffle iron.

2. In the meantime, add the egg in a small mixing bowl and whisk.

3. Add in the ham, cheese, and salt. Mix to combine.

4. Scoop half the mixture using a spoon and pour into the hot waffle iron.

5. Close and cook for 4 minutes.

6. Remove the waffle and place on a large plate. Repeat the process with the remaining batter.

7. In a separate small bowl, add the mayo and mustard. Mix together until smooth.

8. Slice the waffles in quarters and use the mayo mixture as the dip.

303. Cheese-free Breakfast Chaffle

Preparation Time: 4 min
Cooking Time: 12 min
Number of Servings: 1

Ingredients

- 1 egg
- ½ cup almond milk ricotta, finely shredded.
- 1 tbsp almond flour
- 2 tbsp butter

Directions:

1. Mix the egg, almond flour and ricotta in a small bowl.

2. Separate the chaffle batter into two and cook each for 4 minutes.

3. Melt the butter and pour on top of the chaffles.

4. Put them back in the pan and cook on each side for 2 minutes.

5. Remove from the pan and allow them sit for 2 minutes.

6. Enjoy while still crispy.

304. Bacon Chaffle Omelettes

Preparation Time: 5 min
Cooking Time: 10 min
Servings: 2

Ingredients

- 2 slices bacon, raw

- 1 egg
- 1 tsp maple extract, optional
- 1 tsp all spices

Directions:

1. Put the bacon slices in a blender and turn it on.
2. Once ground up, add in the egg and all spices. Go on blending until liquefied.
3. Heat your waffle maker on the highest setting and spray with non-stick cooking spray.
4. Pour half the omelette into the waffle maker and cook for 5 minutes max.
5. Remove the crispy omelette and repeat the same steps with rest batter.
6. Enjoy warm.

305. Avocado Chaffle Toast

Preparation Time: 4 min
Cooking Time: 8 min
Servings: 2

Ingredients

- ½ avocado
- 1 egg
- ½ cup cheddar cheese, finely shredded
- 1 tbsp almond flour
- 1 tsp lemon juice, fresh
- Salt, ground pepper to taste
- Parmesan cheese, finely shredded for garnishing

Directions:

1. Warm up your mini waffle maker.
2. Mix the egg, almond flour with cheese in a small bowl.
3. For a crispy crust, add a teaspoon of

shredded cheese to the waffle maker and cook for 30 seconds.

4. Then, pour the mixture into the waffle maker and cook for 5 minutes or until crispy.
5. Repeat with remaining batter.
6. Mash avocado with a fork until well combined and add lemon juice, salt, pepper
7. Top each chaffle with avocado mixture. Sprinkle with parmesan and enjoy!

306. Crab Chaffles

Preparation Time: 10 min
Cooking Time: 25 min
Servings: 6

Ingredients

- 1 lb crab meat
- 1/3 cup Panko breadcrumbs
- 1 egg
- 2 tbsp fat greek yogurt
- 1 tsp Dijon mustard
- 2 tbsp parsley and chives, fresh
- 1 tsp Italian seasoning
- 1 lemon, juiced
- Salt, pepper to taste

Directions:

1. Preheat the waffle maker
2. Mix all the ingredients in a small mixing bowl, except crab meat.
3. Add the meat. Mix well.
4. Form the mixture into round patties.
5. Cook 1 patty for 3 minutes.
6. Remove it and repeat the process with the remaining crab chaffle mixture.
7. Once ready, remove and enjoy warm.

307. Jalapeno Pepper Chaffle

Preparation time: 10 minutes
Cooking time: 20 minutes
Servings: 4

Ingredients:

- 4 slices of bacon, cooked, crumbled
- 3 tablespoon coconut flour
- 1 jalapeno pepper, deseeded, sliced
- 1 jalapeno pepper, deseeded, diced
- 1 teaspoon baking powder
- ¼ teaspoon of sea salt
- 1 cup / 115 grams shredded cheddar cheese
- 3 eggs, at room temperature
- 1 cup / 225 grams cream cheese, softened

Directions:

1. Take a non-stick waffle iron, plug it in, select the medium or medium-high heat setting and let it preheat until ready to use; it could also be indicated with an indicator light changing its color.

2. Meanwhile, prepare the batter and for this, take a large bowl, add flour in it, stir in baking powder, and salt until mixed.

3. Take another bowl, place cream cheese in it, and beat with an electric mixer until fluffy.

4. Crack eggs in a separate bowl, beat with an electric mixer until fluffy, then add cheddar cheese and ½ cup of beaten cream cheese and continue beating until combined.

5. Add flour mixture into egg-cream cheese mixture, beat with an electric mixer until incorporated, and then fold in diced peppers.

6. Use a ladle to pour one-fourth of the prepared batter into the heated waffle iron in a spiral direction, starting from the edges, then shut the lid and cook for 5 minutes or more until solid and nicely browned; the cooked waffle will look like a cake.

7. When done, transfer chaffles to a plate with a silicone spatula and repeat with the remaining batter.

8. Let chaffles stand for some time until crispy, then top with bacon, jalapeno slices and remaining cream cheese and then serve.

BREAKFAST AND BRUNCH

308.. Avocado Toast Chaffle

Preparation time: 12 minutes
Required cooking time: 6 minutes
Servings available: 2

Ingredients:

- Egg: 2
- Whole avocado: 1 whole
- Salt: ¼ teaspoon or as per your taste
- Cheddar cheese: 1 cup
- Lemon juice: 1 teaspoon
- Black pepper: ¼ teaspoon or as per your taste

Directions:

1. Prepare a mix of peeled and cut avocados into a bowl, add some salt, pepper and lemon juice then mash with a fork. Quickly, preheat a mini-sized waffle and grease it. In another mixing bowl, prepare a mix of cheddar cheese with beaten eggs. Combine the mixture and pour into the lower side of the waffle maker. With the lid closed, cook for 5 minutes to a crunch. Once timed out, take out waffles and allow sitting for a minute. Apply mashed avocado on the chaffles and serve in a plate.

309. Mc Griddle Chaffle

Preparation time: 12 minutes
Required cooking time: 6 minutes
Servings available: 2

Ingredients:

- Egg: 2
- Maple Syrup: 2 tablespoon (sugar-free)
- American cheese: 2 slices
- Swerve/Monk fruit: 2 tablespoon
- Mozzarella Cheese: 1½ cup (shredded)
- Sausage patty: 2

Directions:

1. Quickly preheat a mini-sized waffle maker and grease with oil. Using a mixing bowl, prepare a mix containing shredded mozzarella cheese, beaten eggs, Monk fruit/Swerve and maple syrup and mix into a homogenous state. With a closed lid, heat the waffle for 5 minutes to a crunch. Once timed out, remove the chaffle from the waffle maker. Repeat for the remaining chaffles mixture. Following the instructions on the pack, prepare the sausage patty with a garnish of sliced cheese when removing from heat. Arrange two chaffles with sliced cheese in between and serve hot.

310. Cinnamon Swirl Chaffle

Preparation time: 12 minutes
Required cooking time: 6 minutes
Servings available: 2

Ingredients:

- Icing
- Butter: 2 tablespoons unsalted butter
- Cream cheese: 2 oz softened
- Vanilla: 1 teaspoon
- Splenda: 2 tablespoons
- Chaffle
- Egg: 2
- Almond flour: 2 tablespoons

- Cinnamon: 2 teaspoons
- Splenda: 2 tablespoons
- Cream Cheese: 2 oz softened
- Vanilla Extract: 2 teaspoons
- Vanilla extract: 2 teaspoons
- Cinnamon Drizzle
- Splenda: 2 tablespoons
- Cinnamon: 2 teaspoons
- Butter: 1 tablespoon

Directions:

1. Preheat and grease a waffle maker. Prepare a combined mixture of all ingredients, evenly mixed and pour into the waffle maker. Cook for 4 minutes till chaffles turns crispy, and then set aside. Using a mixing bowl, prepare a mix of all ingredients for icing and the cinnamon drizzle, then heat using a microwave for 12 seconds to soften. Pour heated icing and cinnamon on the cool chaffles to enjoy.

311. Cinnamon Chaffle

Preparation time: 18 minutes
Required cooking time: 12 minutes
Servings available: 2

Ingredients:

- Egg: 1
- Vanilla extract: 1 tablespoon
- Baking powder: ½ teaspoon
- Mozzarella: ½ cup
- Almond flour: 1 tablespoon

Directions:

1. Quickly preheat a mini-sized waffle maker and grease with oil. Using a mixing bowl, prepare a mix containing all the ingredients. With a closed lid, heat the waffle for 5 minutes to a crunch. Once timed out, remove the chaffle from the waffle maker. Repeat for the remaining chaffles mixture. Serve hot with any of your favorite toppings.

312. Japanese Styled Breakfast Chaffle

Preparation time: 12 minutes
Required cooking time: 6 minutes
Servings available: 2

Ingredients:

- Egg: 1
- Bacon: 1 slice
- Green onion: 1 stalk
- Mozzarella Cheese: 1/2 cup (shredded)
- Kewpie Mayo: 2 tablespoon

Directions:

1. Preheat and grease the waffle maker. Using a mixing bowl prepare a mix containing kewpie mayo with beaten egg, then add in ½ chopped green onion with the other ½ kept aside, and ¼ inches of cut bacon into the mixture. Mix evenly. Sprinkle the base of the waffle maker with 1/8 cup of shredded mozzarella and pour in the mixture, then top with more shredded mozzarella. With a closed lid, heat the waffle for 5 minutes to a crunch and then remove the chaffle and allow cooking for a few minutes. Repeat for the remaining chaffles mixture to make more batter. Serve by garnishing the chaffle with the leftover chopped green onions. Enjoy.

313. Keto Strawberry Chaffle

Preparation time:
Cooking time:

Ingredient

- 1 egg
- 1/4 cup mozzarella cheese
- 1 tablespoonful cream cheese
- 1/4 teaspoonful baking powder
- 2 sliced strawberries
- 1 teaspoonfull strawberry extract

Directions:

1. Preheat waffle maker.
2. In a little bowl, beat the egg.
3. Add the rest of the ingredients.
4. The waffle maker is sprayed with non stick cooking spray.
5. Divide the mix into two equal parts.
6. Cook a portion of the mix for around 4 minutes or until golden brown colored.
7. Homemade made whipped cream: 1 cup whipping cream, 1 teaspoonful vanilla, 1 tablespoonful monkfruit confectioners mix. Whip until it forms a mix.

314. Keto Crunchy Chaffle

This sugar-free, without gluten, splendidly firm outwardly, Keto Waffle Recipe can be made instantly with just a blender, a Waffle Iron, and only 5 ingredients! You will be astounded at how great these are.

Preparation time: 15 mins
Cooking time: 8 mins

Ingredients:

- 2 Large Eggs
- 1/2 Cup Shredded Mozarella Cheese (pressed firmly)
- 1/2 teaspoon Baking Powder
- 1 Tablespoon Erythritol (powder), or

sweetener (however powder is most ideal)

- 1/2 teaspoon Vanilla Extract

Driections:

1. Heat You Waffle Iron on the high heat setting. I used a 7 inch waffle Iron and this formula fits nicely for one huge waffle. If you have a smaller waffle iron, you will need to divide the recipe into two waffles.
2. Put all ingredients into a Bullet or a Blender and blend for 10 seconds.
3. Pour the mix into a very hot and dry waffle Iron. It will look thin once poured but have no fear it significantly increases in size when it cooks (and you'll need to keep an eye on it to avoid overflow when cooking!). Let the waffle to Cook for 3-4 minutes or much more! The waffle is done once the entire waffle is golden dark-colored, which takes longer than a normal waffle would. You can use a fork to flip your waffle to ensure that each side has even colors if it doesn't look done after some time. Let waffle cool for 3-4 minutes before eating since it may become brown on cooling
4. Serve with gobs of grass-fed butter and sugar-free syrup, or whatever topping you want.

315. Keto Silver Dollar Pancakes

Preparation time: 10 mins
Cooking time: 5 mins

Ingredients

- (3) Eggs
- 1/2 Cup (105 G) Cottage Cheese
- 1/3 Cup (37.33 G) Superfine Almond Flour

- 1/4 Cup (62.5 G) Unsweetened Almond Milk
- 2 Tablespoons Truvia
- Vanilla Extract
- 1 Teaspoon Baking Powder
- Cooking Oil Spray

Directions:

1. place ingredients in a blender in the order listed above. Mix until you have a smooth, fluid batter.

2. Heat a nonstick pan on medium-high temperature. Spray with oil or margarine.

3. Place 2 tablespoons of batter at once to make little, dollar hotcakes. This is an extremely fluid, sensitive batter so don't

4. attempt to make big pancakes with this one as they won't flip over easily.

5. Cook every pancake until the top of the hotcake has made little air pockets and the air pockets have vanished, around 1-2 minutes.

6. Using a spatula, tenderly loosen the pan cake, and afterward flip over.

7. Make the remainder of the pancakes and serve hot.

316. Keto Chaffle Waffle

Preparation time:
Cooking time:

Ingredients:

- 1 egg
- ½ cup of shredded mozzarella cheese
- 1 ½ table-spoon of almond flour
- Pinch of baking powder
- Equipment:
- Waffle Maker

- Shredder (to shred solid mozzarella cheese)

Directions:

1. Start by turning your waffle maker on and preheating it. During the time of pre-heating, in a bowl, whisk the egg and shredded mozzarella cheese together. If you do not have shredded mozzarella cheese, you can use the shredder to shred your cheese, Then add the almond powder and baking powder to the bowl and whisk them until the mixture is consistent.

2. Then pour the mixture onto the waffle machine. Make sure you pour it to the center of the mixture will come out of the edges on closing the machine. Close the machine and let the waffles cook until golden brown. Then you can serve your tasty chaffle waffles.

Nutrition:

Serves 1 person
Calories 320
Carbohydrates 2.9 g
Protein 21.5 g
Fat 24.3g

317. Keto Chaffle Topped With Salted Caramel Syrup

Preparation time: 15 mins
Cooking time: 10 mins

Ingredients:

- 1 egg
- ½ cup of mozzarella cheese
- ¼ cup of cream
- 2 tablespoon of collagen powder
- 1 ½ tablespoon of almond flour
- 1 ½ tablespoon of unsalted butter
- Pinch of salt

- ¾ tablespoon of powdered erythritol
- Pinch of baking powder

Directions:

1. Begin by preheating your waffle machine by switching it on and turning the heat to medium. Whisk together the chaffle ingredients that include the egg, mozzarella cheese, almond flour, and baking powder. Pour the mixture on the waffle machine. Let it cook until golden brown. You can make up to two chaffles with this method.

2. To make the caramel syrup, you will need to turn on the flame under a pan to medium heat Melt the unsalted butter on the pan. Then turn the heat low and add collagen powder and erythritol to the pan and whisk them. Gradually add the cream and remove from heat. Then add the salt and continue to whisk. Pour the syrup onto the chaffle, and here you go.

Nutrition:

1 serving
605 calories
45g fat
48g protein
g of carbohydrates

318. Keto Chaffle Bacon Sandwich

Preparation time: 15 mins
Cooking time: 10 mins

Ingredients:

- 1 egg
- ½ cup of shredded mozzarella cheese
- 2 Tablespoon of coconut flour
- 2 strips of pork or beef bacon
- 1 slice of any type of cheese
- 2 tablespoon of coconut oil

Directions:

1. To make the chaffle, you will be following the typical recipe for making a chaffle. Start by warming your waffle machine to medium heat. In a bowl, beat 1 egg, ½ cup of mozzarella cheese, and almond flour. Pour the mixture on the waffle machine. Let it cook until it is golden brown. Then remove in a plate.

2. Warm coconut oil in a pan over medium heat. Then place the bacon strips in the pan. Cook until crispy over medium heat. Assemble the bacon and cheese on the chaffle.

Nutrition:

Serving size 1
Calories 580
Fat 52 g
Carbohydrates 3g

319. Crispy Zucchini Chaffle

Preparation time: 15 mins
Cooking time: 5 mins

Ingredients:

- 2 eggs
- 1 fresh zucchini
- 1 cup of shredded or grated cheddar cheese
- 2 pinch of salt
- 1 tablespoon of onion (chopped)
- 1 clove of garlic

Directions:

1. Start by preheating the waffle maker to medium heat. The best way to make a chaffle is to make it with layering. Start by dicing onions and mashing the garlic. Then use the grater to grate the zucchini. Then take a bowl and add 2 eggs and add the

grated zucchini to the bowl.

2. Also, add the onions, salt, and garlic for extra flavor. You can also add other herbs to give your zaffle a crispy more flavor. Then sprinkle ½ cup of cheese on top of the waffle machine.

3. Add the mixture from the bowl to the waffle machine. Add the remaining cheese on top of the waffle machine and close the waffle machine. Make sure the waffle cooks for about 3 to 5 minutes until it turns golden brown.

4. By the layering method, you will achieve the perfect crisp. Take out your zucchini chaffles and serve them hot and fresh.

5. Equipment:

6. Waffle maker

7. Grater to grate the cheese

Nutrition:

Serving size 2
Calories 170
Fat 12g
Carbohydrates 4g
Protein 11g

320. Peanut Butter Chaffle

Preparation time: 15 min
Cooking time: 10 min

Ingredients:

- 1 egg

- ½ cup of cheddar cheese

- 2 tablespoon of peanut butter

- Few drops of vanilla extract

Directions:

1. To make deliciously tasting peanut butter chaffles. Take a grater and grate some cheddar cheese. Add one egg, cheddar cheese, 2 tablespoon of

peanut butter, and a few drops of vanilla extract. Beat these ingredients together until the batter is consistent enough.

2. Then sprinkle some shredded cheese as a base on the waffle maker. Pour the mixture on top of the waffle machine.

3. Sprinkle more cheese on top of the mixture and close the waffle machine. Ensure that the waffle is cooked thoroughly for about a few minutes until they are golden brown. Then remove it and enjoy your deliciously cooked chaffles.

Equipment:

Waffle maker

Grater

Nutrition:

1 serving
363 Calories
29 g of Fat
22 g of Protein
4 g of Carbohydrates

321. Morning Chaffles With Berries

Preparation Time: 5 Min
Cooking Time: 5 Min
Servings: 4

Ingredients

- 1 Cup Egg Whites

- 1 cup cheddar cheese, shredded

- ¼ cup almond flour

- ¼ cup heavy cream

Topping

- 4 Oz. Raspberries

- 4 Oz. Strawberries.

- 1 Oz. Keto Chocolate Flakes

- 1 Oz. Feta Cheese.

Directions

1. Preheat your square waffle maker and grease with cooking spray.
2. Beat egg white in a small bowl with flour.
3. Add shredded cheese to the egg whites and flour mixture and mix well.
4. Add cream and cheese tothe egg mixture.
5. Pour Chaffles batter in a waffle maker and close the lid.
6. Cook chaffles for about 4 minutes until crispy and brown.
7. Carefully remove chaffles from the maker.
8. Serve with berries, cheese, and chocolate on top.
9. Enjoy!

322. Chaffles Breakfast Bowl

Preparation Time: 10 Min
Cooking Time: 5 Min
Servings: 2

Ingredients

- 1 Egg
- 1/2 cup cheddar cheese shredded
- pinch of Italian seasoning
- 1 tbsp. pizza sauce

Topping

- 1/2 Avocado Sliced
- 2 Eggs Boiled
- 1 Tomato, Halves
- 4 Oz. Fresh Spinach Leaves

Directions

1. Preheat yourwaffle maker and grease with cooking spray.
2. Crack an egg in a small bowl and beat with Italian seasoning and pizza sauce.
3. Add shredded cheese to the egg and spices mixture.
4. Pour 1 tbsp. shredded cheese in a waffle maker and cook for 30 sec.
5. Pour Chaffles batter inthe waffle maker and close the lid.
6. Cook chaffles for about 4 minutes until crispy and brown.
7. Carefully remove chaffles from the maker.
8. Serve on the bed of spinach with boil egg, avocado slice, and tomatoes.
9. Enjoy!

323. Crispy Chaffles With Sausage

Preparation Time: 5 Min
Cooking Time: 10 Min
Servings: 2

Ingredients

- 1/2 cup cheddar cheese
- 1/2 tsp. baking powder
- 1/4 cup egg whites
- 2 tsp. pumpkin spice
- 1 egg, whole
- 2 chicken sausage
- 2 slice bacon
- salt and pepper to taste
- 1 tsp. avocado oil

Directions:

1. Mix together all ingredients in a bowl.
2. Allow batter to sit while waffle iron warms.

3. Spray waffle iron with nonstick spray.

4. Pour batter in the waffle maker and cook according to the directions of the manufacturer.

5. Meanwhile, heat oil in a pan and fry the egg, according to your choice and transfer it toa plate.

6. In the same pan, fry bacon slice and sausage on medium heat for about 2-3 minutes until cooked.

7. Once chaffles are cooked thoroughly, remove them from the maker.

8. Serve with fried egg, bacon slice, sausages and enjoy!

324. Mini Breakfast Chaffles

Preparation Time: 5 Min
Cooking Time: 15 Min
Servings: 3

Ingredients

- 6 tsp coconut flour
- 1 tsp stevia
- 1/4 tsp baking powder
- 2 eggs
- 3 oz. cream cheese
- 1/2. tsp vanilla extract

Topping

- 1 egg
- 6 slice bacon
- 2 oz. Raspberries for topping
- 2 oz. Blueberries for topping
- 2 oz. Strawberries for topping

Directions:

1. Heat up your square waffle maker and grease with cooking spray.

2. Mix together coconut flour, stevia, egg,

baking powder, cheese and vanilla in mixing bowl.

3. Pour ½ of chaffles mixture in a waffle maker.

4. Close the lid and cook the chaffles for about 3-5 minutes.

5. Meanwhile, fry bacon slices in pan on medium heat for about 2-3 minutes until cooked and transfer themto plate.

6. In the same pan, fry eggs one by one in the leftover grease of bacon.

7. Once chaffles are cooked, carefully transferthem toplate.

8. Serve with fried eggs and bacon slice and berries on top.

9. Enjoy!

325. Crispy Chaffles With Egg & Asparagus

Preparation Time: 5 Min
Cooking Time: 10 Min
Servings: 1

Ingredients

- 1 egg
- 1/4 cup cheddar cheese
- 2 tbsps. almond flour
- ½ tsp. baking powder

TOPPING

- 1 egg
- 4-5 stalks asparagus
- 1 tsp avocado oil

Directions:

1. Preheat waffle maker to medium-high heat.

2. Whisk together egg, mozzarella cheese, almond flour, and baking

powder

3. Pour chaffles mixture into the center of the waffle iron. Close the waffle maker and let cook for 3-5 minutes or until waffle is golden brown and set.

4. Remove chaffles from the waffle maker and serve.

5. Meanwhile, heat oil in a nonstick pan.

6. Once the pan is hot, fry asparagus for about 4-5 minutes until golden brown.

7. Poach the egg in boil water for about 2-3 minutes.

8. Once chaffles are cooked, remove from the maker.

9. Serve chaffles with the poached egg and asparagus.

326. Coconut Chaffles

Preparation Time: 5 Min
Cooking Time: 5 Min
Servings: 2

Ingredients

- 1 egg
- 1 oz. cream cheese,
- 1 oz. cheddar cheese
- 2 tbsps. coconut flour
- 1 tsp. stevia
- 1 tbsp. coconut oil, melted
- 1/2 tsp. coconut extract
- 2 eggs, soft boil for serving

Directions:

1. Heat you mini Dash waffle maker and grease with cooking spray.

2. Mix together all chaffles ingredients in a bowl.

3. Pour chaffle batter in a preheated waffle maker.

4. Close the lid.

5. Cook chaffles for about 2-3 minutes until golden brown.

6. Serve with boil egg and enjoy!

327. Raspberry-Yogurt Chaffle Bowl

Preparation time: 10 minutes
Cooking time: 14 minutes
Servings: 2

Ingredients:

- 1 egg, beaten
- 1 tbsp almond flour
- ¼ cup finely grated mozzarella cheese
- ¼ tsp baking powder
- 1 cup Greek yogurt
- 1 cup fresh raspberries
- 2 tbsp almonds, chopped

Directions:

1. Preheat a waffle bowl maker and grease lightly with cooking spray.

2. Meanwhile, in a medium bowl, whisk all the ingredients except the yogurt, raspberries until smooth batter forms.

3. Open the iron, pour in half of the mixture, cover, and cook until crispy, 6 to 7 minutes.

4. Remove the chaffle bowl onto a plate and set aside.

5. Make the second chaffle bowl with the remaining batter.

6. To serve, divide the yogurt into the chaffle bowls and top with the raspberries and almonds.

328. Bacon-Cheddar Biscuit Chaffle

Preparation time: 10 minutes
Cooking time: 28 minutes

Servings: 4

Ingredients:

- 1 egg, beaten
- 2 tbsp almond flour
- 2 tbsp ground flaxseed
- 3 bacon slices, cooked and chopped
- ¼ cup heavy cream
- 1 ½ tbsp melted butter
- ½ cup finely grated Gruyere cheese
- ½ cup finely grated cheddar cheese
- ¼ tsp erythritol
- ½ tsp onion powder
- ½ tsp garlic salt
- ½ tbsp dried parsley
- ½ tbsp baking powder
- ¼ tsp baking soda

Directions:

1. Preheat the waffle iron.
2. Meanwhile, in a medium bowl, whisk all the ingredients until smooth batter forms.
3. Open the iron, pour a quarter of the mixture into the iron, close and cook until crispy, 6 to 7 minutes.
4. Remove the chaffle onto a plate and set aside.
5. Make three more Chaffles with the remaining batter.
6. Allow cooling and serve afterward.

329. Turnip Hash Brown Chaffles

Preparation time: 10 minutes
Cooking time: 42 minutes
Servings: 6

Ingredients:

- 1 large turnip, peeled and shredded
- ½ medium white onion, minced
- 2 garlic cloves, pressed
- 1 cup finely grated Gouda cheese
- 2 eggs, beaten
- Salt and freshly ground black pepper to taste

Directions:

1. Pour the turnips in a medium safe microwave bowl, sprinkle with 1 tbsp of water, and steam in the microwave until softened, 1 to 2 minutes.
2. Remove the bowl and mix in the remaining ingredients except for a quarter cup of the Gouda cheese.
3. Preheat the waffle iron.
4. Once heated, open and sprinkle some of the reserved cheese in the iron and top with 3 tablespoons of the mixture. Close the waffle iron and cook until crispy, 5 minutes.
5. Open the lid, flip the chaffle and cook further for 2 more minutes.
6. Remove the chaffle onto a plate and set aside.
7. Make five more chaffles with the remaining batter in the same proportion.
8. Allow cooling and serve afterward.

330. Everything Bagel Chaffles

Preparation time: 10 minutes
Cooking time: 28 minutes
Servings: 4

Ingredients:

- 1 egg, beaten
- ½ cup finely grated Parmesan cheese
- 1 tsp Everything Bagel seasoning

Directions:

1. Preheat the waffle iron.

2. In a medium bowl, mix all the ingredients.

3. Open the iron, pour in a quarter of the mixture, close, and cook until crispy, 6 to 7 minutes.

4. Remove the chaffle onto a plate and set aside.

5. Make three more chaffles, allow cooling, and enjoy after.

331. Blueberry Shortcake Chaffles

Preparation time: 10 minutes
Cooking time: 14 minutes
Servings: 2

Ingredients:

- 1 egg, beaten
- 1 tbsp cream cheese, softened
- ¼ cup finely grated mozzarella cheese
- 1/4 tsp baking powder
- 4 fresh blueberries
- 1 tsp blueberry extract

Directions:

1. Preheat the waffle iron.

2. In a medium bowl, mix all the ingredients.

3. Open the iron, pour in half of the batter, close, and cook until crispy, 6 to 7 minutes.

4. Remove the chaffle onto a plate and set aside.

5. Make the other chaffle with the remaining batter.

6. Allow cooling and enjoy after.

332. Raspberry-Pecan Chaffles

Preparation time: 10 minutes
Cooking time: 14 minutes
Servings: 2

Ingredients:

- 1 egg, beaten
- ½ cup finely grated mozzarella cheese
- 1 tbsp cream cheese, softened
- 1 tbsp sugar-free maple syrup
- ¼ tsp raspberry extract
- ¼ tsp vanilla extract
- 2 tbsp sugar-free caramel sauce for topping
- 3 tbsp chopped pecans for topping

Directions:

1. Preheat the waffle iron.

2. In a medium bowl, mix all the ingredients.

3. Open the iron, pour in half of the batter, close, and cook until crispy, 6 to 7 minutes.

4. Remove the chaffle onto a plate and set aside.

5. Make another chaffle with the remaining batter.

6. To serve: drizzle the caramel sauce on the chaffles and top with the pecans.

333. Breakfast Spinach Ricotta Chaffles

Preparation time: 10 minutes
Cooking time: 28 minutes
Servings: 4

Ingredients:

- 4 oz frozen spinach, thawed, squeezed dry
- 1 cup ricotta cheese
- 2 eggs, beaten

- ½ tsp garlic powder
- ¼ cup finely grated Pecorino Romano cheese
- ½ cup finely grated mozzarella cheese
- Salt and freshly ground black pepper to taste

Directions:

1. Preheat the waffle iron.
2. In a medium bowl, mix all the ingredients.
3. Open the iron, lightly grease with cooking spray and spoon in a quarter of the mixture.
4. Close the iron and cook until brown and crispy, 7 minutes.
5. Remove the chaffle onto a plate and set aside.
1. Make three more chaffles with the remaining mixture.
2. Allow cooling and serve afterward.

334. Scrambled Egg Stuffed Chaffles

Preparation time: 15 minutes
Cooking time: 28 minutes
Servings: 4

Ingredients:

- For the chaffles:
- 1 cup finely grated cheddar cheese
- 2 eggs, beaten
- For the egg stuffing:
- 1 tbsp olive oil
- 4 large eggs
- 1 small green bell pepper, deseeded and chopped
- 1 small red bell pepper, deseeded and chopped
- Salt and freshly ground black pepper

to taste
- 2 tbsp grated Parmesan cheese

Directions:

1. For the chaffles:
2. Preheat the waffle iron.
3. In a medium bowl, mix the cheddar cheese and egg.
4. Open the iron, pour in a quarter of the mixture, close, and cook until crispy, 6 to 7 minutes.
5. Plate and make three more chaffles using the remaining mixture.
6. For the egg stuffing:
7. Meanwhile, heat the olive oil in a medium skillet over medium heat on a stovetop.
8. In a medium bowl, beat the eggs with the bell peppers, salt, black pepper, and Parmesan cheese.
9. Pour the mixture into the skillet and scramble until set to your likeness, 2 minutes.
10. Between two chaffles, spoon half of the scrambled eggs and repeat with the second set of chaffles.
01. Serve afterward.

335. Mixed Berry-Vanilla Chaffles

Preparation time: 10 minutes
Cooking time: 28 minutes
Servings: 4

Ingredients:

- 1 egg, beaten
- ½ cup finely grated mozzarella cheese
- 1 tbsp cream cheese, softened
- 1 tbsp sugar-free maple syrup
- 2 strawberries, sliced

- 2 raspberries, slices
- ¼ tsp blackberry extract
- ¼ tsp vanilla extract
- ½ cup plain yogurt for serving

Directions:

1. Preheat the waffle iron.
2. In a medium bowl, mix all the ingredients except the yogurt.
3. Open the iron, lightly grease with cooking spray and pour in a quarter of the mixture.
4. Close the iron and cook until golden brown and crispy, 7 minutes.
5. Remove the chaffle onto a plate and set aside.
6. Make three more chaffles with the remaining mixture.
7. To serve: top with the yogurt and enjoy.

336. Ham and Cheddar Chaffles

Preparation time: 15 minutes
Cooking time: 28 minutes
Servings: 4

Ingredients:

- 1 cup finely shredded parsnips, steamed
- 8 oz ham, diced
- 2 eggs, beaten
- 1 ½ cups finely grated cheddar cheese
- ½ tsp garlic powder
- 2 tbsp chopped fresh parsley leaves
- ¼ tsp smoked paprika
- ½ tsp dried thyme
- Salt and freshly ground black pepper to taste

Directions:

1. Preheat the waffle iron.
2. In a medium bowl, mix all the ingredients.
3. Open the iron, lightly grease with cooking spray and pour in a quarter of the mixture.
4. Close the iron and cook until crispy, 7 minutes.
5. Remove the chaffle onto a plate and set aside.
6. Make three more chaffles using the remaining mixture.
7. Serve afterward.

337. Savory Gruyere and Chives Chaffles

Preparation time: 15 minutes
Cooking time: 14 minutes
Servings: 2

Ingredients:

- 2 eggs, beaten
- 1 cup finely grated Gruyere cheese
- 2 tbsp finely grated cheddar cheese
- 1/8 tsp freshly ground black pepper
- 3 tbsp minced fresh chives + more for garnishing
- 2 sunshine fried eggs for topping

Directions:

1. Preheat the waffle iron.
2. In a medium bowl, mix the eggs, cheeses, black pepper, and chives.
3. Open the iron and pour in half of the mixture.
4. Close the iron and cook until brown and crispy, 7 minutes.
5. Remove the chaffle onto a plate and

set aside.

6. Make another chaffle using the remaining mixture.

7. Top each chaffle with one fried egg each, garnish with the chives and serve.

338. Chicken Quesadilla Chaffle

Preparation time: 10 minutes
Cooking time: 14 minutes
Servings: 2

Ingredients:

- 1 egg, beaten
- ¼ tsp taco seasoning
- 1/3 cup finely grated cheddar cheese
- 1/3 cup cooked chopped chicken

Directions:

1. Preheat the waffle iron.

2. In a medium bowl, mix the eggs, taco seasoning, and cheddar cheese. Add the chicken and combine well.

3. Open the iron, lightly grease with cooking spray and pour in half of the mixture.

4. Close the iron and cook until brown and crispy, 7 minutes.

5. Remove the chaffle onto a plate and set aside.

6. Make another chaffle using the remaining mixture.

7. Serve afterward.

339. Hot Chocolate Breakfast Chaffle

Preparation time: 10 minutes
Cooking time: 14 minutes
Servings: 2

Ingredients:

- 1 egg, beaten
- 2 tbsp almond flour
- 1 tbsp unsweetened cocoa powder
- 2 tbsp cream cheese, softened
- ¼ cup finely grated Monterey Jack cheese
- 2 tbsp sugar-free maple syrup
- 1 tsp vanilla extract

Directions:

1. Preheat the waffle iron.

2. In a medium bowl, mix all the ingredients.

3. Open the iron, lightly grease with cooking spray and pour in half of the mixture.

4. Close the iron and cook until crispy, 7 minutes.

5. Remove the chaffle onto a plate and set aside.

6. Pour the remaining batter in the iron and make the second chaffle.

7. Allow cooling and serve afterward.

LUNCH AND DINNER RECIPES

340. Chicken Cauli Chaffle

Preparation time: 27 minutes
Required cooking time: 12 minutes
Servings: 2

Ingredients:

- Chicken: 3-4 pieces or ½ cup when done
- Garlic: 2 cloves (finely grated)
- Egg: 2
- Salt: As per your taste
- Green onion: 1 stalk
- Soy Sauce: 1 tablespoon
- Cauliflower Rice: 1 cup
- Mozzarella cheese: 1 cup
- Black pepper: ¼ teaspoon or as per your taste
- White pepper: ¼ teaspoon or as per your taste

Directions:

1. Melt some butter in an oven and set aside, then cook the chicken in a skillet using salt and a cup of water to boil. With the lid closed, cook for 18 minutes. Once done, put off the heat and shred the chicken into pieces, then discard all bones.

2. Using another mixing bowl prepare a mix containing peppers (white and black), soy sauce, cauliflower rice, grated garlic, beaten egg with the shredded chicken pieces. Mix evenly. Preheat and grease the waffle maker. Pour 1/8 cup of mozzarella into the waffle maker with the mixture on the cheese, add another cup (1/8) of mozzarella on the chaffle. With a closed lid, heat the waffle for 5 minutes to a crunch and then remove the chaffle. Repeat for the remaining chaffles mixture to make more batter. Serve by garnishing the chaffle with chopped green onions and enjoy.

341. Garlic Chicken Chaffle

Preparation time: 27 minutes
Required cooking time: 12 minutes
Servings: 2

Ingredients:

- Chicken: 3-4 pieces
- Garlic: 1 clove
- Egg: 1
- Salt
- Lemon juice: ½ tablespoon
- Kewpie mayo: 2 tablespoon
- Mozzarella cheese: ½ cup

Directions:

1. Cook the chicken in a skillet using salt and a cup of water to boil. With the lid closed, cook for 18 minutes. Once done, put off the heat and shred the chicken into pieces, then discard all bones. Using another mixing bowl prepare a mix containing 1/8 cup of cheese, Kewpie mayo, lemon juice and grated garlic. Mix evenly. Preheat and grease the waffle maker. Arrange chaffles on a baking tray with the chicken, then sprinkle cheese on the chaffles. With a closed lid, heat the waffle for 5 minutes until cheese melts and then remove the chaffle. Repeat for the remaining chaffles mixture to make more batter. Serve and warm.

342. Buffalo Chicken Chaffle

Preparation time: 12 minutes
Required cooking time: 6 minutes
Servings: 2

Ingredients:

- Egg: 2

- Buffalo sauce: 4 tablespoons (can be as desired)

- Chicken: 1 cup

- Cheddar Cheese: 1 cup

- Softened cream cheese: ¼ cup

- Butter: 1 teaspoon

Directions:

1. Melt some butter in a pan with shredded chicken added into it. Add tablespoons of buffalo sauce into the heated mix. Using a mixing bowl, prepare a mixture containing eggs with whipped cream cheese, cheddar cheese and cooked chicken, then mix evenly. Preheat and grease a waffle maker. Sprinkle some cheddar cheese at the base of the waffle maker, then the mixture spread evenly on the waffle maker with a bit of cheese. Heat to a crispy form for 5 minutes and repeat the process for the remaining batter. Serve the dish with some buffalo sauce to enjoy.

343. Chicken Mozzarella Chaffle

Preparation time: 12 minutes
Required cooking time: 6 minutes
Servings: 2

Ingredients:

- Chicken: 1 cup

- Mozzarella cheese: 1 cup and 4 tablespoons

- Basil: ½ teaspoon

- Butter: 1 teaspoon

- Egg: 2

- Tomato sauce: 6 tablespoons

- Garlic: ½ tablespoon

Directions:

1. Melt some butter in a pan with shredded chicken added into it and stir for few minutes. Add basil with garlic and set aside. Using a mixing bowl, prepare a mixture containing eggs with cooked chicken and mozzarella cheese, then mix evenly. Preheat and grease a waffle maker. Spread the mixture on the base of the mini-waffle maker evenly, then heat for 5 minutes to a crispy form. Repeat the process for the remaining batter. On a baking tray, arrange the chaffles with tomato sauce and grated cheese to garnish the top. Heat the oven at 399F to melt cheese then serve best hot.

344 Chicken Bbq Chaffle

Preparation time: 32 minutes
Required cooking time: 11 minutes
Servings: 2

Ingredients:

- Chicken: 1/2 cup

- BBQ sauce: 1 tablespoon (sugar-free)

- Egg: 1

- Almond flour: 2 tablespoon

- Cheddar cheese: ½ cup

- Butter: 1 tablespoon

Directions:

1. Melt some butter in a pan with shredded chicken added into it and stir for 11 minutes. Using a mixing bowl, prepare a mixture containing all ingredients with the cooked chicken, then mix evenly.

Preheat and grease a waffle maker. Spread the mixture on the base of the waffle maker evenly, and then heat for 7 minutes to a crispy form. Repeat the process for the remaining batter. Serve best hot.

345. Chicken Spinach Chaffle

Preparation time: 41 minutes
Required cooking time: 11 minutes
Servings: 2

Ingredients:

- Spinach: ½ cup
- Pepper: As per your taste
- Basil: 1 teaspoon
- Chicken: ½ cup boneless
- Shredded mozzarella: half cup
- Garlic powder: 1 tablespoon
- Salt: As per your taste
- Egg: 1
- Onion powder: 1 tablespoon

Directions:

1. Heat the chicken in water to boil, then shred it into pieces and keep aside. Heat the spinach for 9 minutes to strain. Using a mixing bowl, prepare a mixture containing all ingredients with the cooked chicken, then mix evenly. Preheat and grease a waffle maker. Spread the mixture on the base of the waffle maker evenly, and then heat for 7 minutes to a crispy form. Repeat the process for the remaining batter. Serve best crispy with your desired keto sauce.

346. Chicken Parmesan Chaffle

Preparation time: 30 mins
Cooking time: 5 mins

Ingredients

- 1/2 Cup Canned Chicken Breast Or Leftover Shredded Chicken
- 1/4 Cup Cheddar Cheese
- 1/8 Cup Parmesan Cheese
- 1 Egg
- 1 Teaspoon Italian Seasoning
- 1/8 Teaspoon Garlic Powder
- 1 Teaspoon Cream Cheese, Room Temperature
- Topping Ingredients
- 2 Slices Of Provolone Cheese
- 1 Tablespoon Sugar-Free Pizza Sauce I Like Using Rao's Sauces!

Directions:

1. Preheat the mini waffle maker.
2. In a medium-size bowl, add all the ingredients and mix until it's fully incorporated.
3. Add a teaspoon of shredded cheese to the waffle iron for 30 seconds before adding the mixture.
4. This will create the best crust and make it easier to take this heavy chaffle out of the waffle maker when it's done.
5. Pour half of the mixture in the mini waffle maker and cook it for a minimum of 4 to 5 minutes.
6. Repeat the above steps to cook the second Chicken Parmesan Chaffle.
7. Top with a sugar-free pizza sauce and one slice of provolone cheese. I like to sprinkle the top with even more Italian Seasoning too!

347. Corndog Chaffle

Preparation time: 45 mins
Cooking time: 5 mins

Ingredients

- 2 Eggs
- 1 Cup Mexican Cheese Blend
- 1 Tablespoon Almond Flour
- 1/2 Teaspoon Cornbread Extract
- 1/4 Teaspoon Salt
- Hot Dogs With Hot Dog Sticks
- Optional: For Extra Added Spice Be Sure To Add Diced Jalapenos To This Recipe!

Directions:

1. Preheat corndog waffle maker.
2. In a small bowl, whip the eggs.
3. Add the remaining ingredients, except for the hotdogs
4. Spray the corndog waffle maker with non-stick cooking spray.
5. Fill the corndog waffle maker with the batter halfway filled. (if you want a crispy corndog, add a small amount of cheese 30 seconds before adding the batter)
6. Place a stick in the hot dog.
7. Place the hot dog in the batter and slightly press down.
8. Spread a small amount of batter on top of the hot dog, just enough to fill it.
9. Makes about 4 to 5 chaffle corndogs
10. Cook the corndog chaffles for about 4 minutes or until golden brown.
11. When done, they will easily remove from the corndog waffle maker with a pair of tongs.
12. Serve with mustard, mayo, or sugar-free ketchup!

348. Burger Bun Chaffle

Preparation time: 3 mins
Cooking time: 5 mins

Ingredients

- 1 Large Egg, Beaten
- 1/2 Cup Shredded Mozzarella
- 1 Tb Almond Flour
- 1/4 Tsp Baking Powder
- 1 Teaspoon Sesame Seeds
- 1 Pinch Of Onion Powder

Directions

1. Combine all ingredients
2. Pour half into a mini waffle maker (or split between two)
3. Cook for 5 minutes or until you no longer see steam coming from the waffle maker.
4. Remove to a wire rack and allow to cool.

349. Halloumi Cheese Chaffle

Preparation time: 5 mins
Cooking time: 5 mins

Ingredients

- 3 Ounces Halloumi Cheese
- 2 Tablespoons Pasta Sauce Optional

Directions:

1. Cut Halloumi cheese into 1/2 inch thick slices.
2. Place cheese in the UNHEATED waffle maker.
3. Turn waffle maker on.
4. Let it cook for about 3-6 minutes or until golden brown and to your liking.
5. Let it cool for some time on a rack.

6. Add Low Carb marinara or pasta sauce.

7. Serve immediately. Enjoy!

350. Keto Sausage Ball Chaffle Recipe

Preparation Time: 10mins
Cooking Time: 5mins
Serving: 3

Ingredients

- 1 Pound Bulk Italian
- 1 Cup Sharp Cheddar
- Sausage
- Cheese
- 1 Cup Almond Flour
- 1/4 Cup Parmesan
- 2 Tsp Baking Powder
- Cheese
- 1 Egg

Directions:

1. Preheat the smaller than normal Chaffle producer.

2. Consolidate all ingredient in an enormous blending bowl and blend well utilizing your hands.

3. Spot a paper plate under Chaffle creator to get any spillage.

4. Scoop 3 T of blend onto warmed Chaffle creator.

5. Cook for at least 3 minutes. Flip over and cook 2

6. additional minutes for even firmness.

351. Pumpkin Cake Chaffle

Preparation Time: 10mins
Cooking Time: 10mins
Serving: 4

Ingredients

- 1 Egg
- Frosting
- 1/2 Cup Mozzarella
- Ingredients:
- Cheese
- 2 Tbs Cream Cheese
- 1/2 Tsp Pumpkin Pie
- 2 Tbs Monkfruit
- Spice
- Confectioners Blend
- 1 Tbs Pumpkin
- 1/2 Tsp Clear Vanilla
- Extract

Directions:

1. Preheat the little Chaffle producer. In a little bowl, whip the egg.

2. Include the cheddar, pumpkin pie flavor, and the pumpkin.

3. Include 1/2 of the blend to the little Chaffle producer and cook it for at any rate 3 to 4 minutes until it's brilliant darker.

4. While the chaffle is cooking, include the entirety of the cream cheddar icing ingredients in a bowl and blend it until it's smooth and rich.

5. On the off chance that you need a rich taste to this icing, you can likewise include a tbs of genuine margarine that has been relaxed at room

6. temperature.

7. Add the cream cheddar icing to the hot chaffle and serve it right away.

352. Keto Lemon Chaffle Recipe

Preparation Time: 10mins
Cooking Time: 10mins
Serving: 4

Ingredients

- Chaffle Cake:
- 20 Drops Cake
- 2- Oz Cream Cheese
- Batter Extract
- 2 Eggs
- Chaffle Frosting:
- 2 Tsp Butter
- 1/2 Cup Heavy
- 2 Tbs Coconut Flour
- Whipping Cream
- 1 Tsp Monkfruit
- 1 Tbs Monkfruit
- 1 Tsp Baking Powder
- 1/4 Tsp Lemon
- 1/2 Tsp Lemon
- Extract
- Extract

Directions:

1. Preheat the smaller than normal Chaffle producer 67

2. Include the entirety of the elements for the chaffle cake in a blender and blend it until the hitter is decent and smooth. This should just take a few minutes.

3. Utilize a dessert scoop and fill the Chaffle iron with one full scoop of hitter. This size of the frozen yogurt scoop is around 3 tsp and fits superbly in the smaller than usual Chaffle producer.

4. While the chaffles are cooking, start making the icing.

5. In a medium-size bowl, include the chaffle icing ingredients.

6. Blend the ingredients until the icing is thick with tops. All the chaffles to totally cool before icing the cake

7. Discretionary: Add lemon strip for additional flavor!

353. Cinnamon Roll Chaffles

Preparation Time: 5mins
Cooking Time: 15mins
Serving: 2

Ingredients

- 2- large eggs
- 1/2 tsp. kosher salt
- 2- tbsp. almond
- 1/2- tsp. baking
- flour
- soda
- tsp. pure vanilla
- c. shredded
- extract
- mozzarella
- tbsp. granulated
- Cooking spray:
- swerve
- oz. cream cheese
- 1/2- tsp. cinnamon
- tbsp. heavy cream

Directions:

1. Preheat Chaffle iron to high. In an enormous bowl, beat eggs. Mix in almond flour, vanilla, 1 tsp 69

2. swerve, cinnamon, salt, and preparing

pop. Toss in mozzarella.

3. Oil Chaffle iron with cooking shower, at that point Pour portion of the hitter into the Chaffle iron and cook until light brilliant, around 3 minutes.

4. Rehash with the outstanding hitter.

5. In a medium microwave-safe bowl, join cream cheddar, substantial cream, and staying 1 tsp swerve. Microwave, whisking like clockwork, until softened and drizzly

6. Top Chaffles with strawberries and sprinkle with cream cheddar blend and maple syrup.

354. Keto Cheese Chaffle Recipe

Preparation Time: 10mins
Cooking Time: 8mins
Serving: 2

Ingredients

- 1 large egg
- 1/2 c. shredded cheese
- Pinch of salt
- Seasoning

Directions:

1. Preheat the scaled-down Chaffle producer, in a bowl, whisk the egg until beaten.

2. Shred the cheddar

3. Include the cheddar, salt, and flavoring to the egg, at that point blend well.

4. Scoop half of the blend on the Chaffle producer spread uniformly.

5. Cook 3-4 minutes, until done exactly as you would prefer, pull it off and let cool.

6. Include the remainder of the hitter and cook the second Chaffle.

7. Enjoy

355. Maple Pumpkin Keto Chaffle Recipe

Preparation Time: 5mins
Cooking Time: 16mins
Servings: 2

Ingredients

- 2 eggs
- 2 tsp Lakanto
- 3/4 tsp baking
- Sugar-Free Maple
- powder
- Syrup
- 2 tsp pumpkin
- 1 tsp coconut flour
- puree
- 1/2 cup mozzarella
- 3/4 tsp pumpkin
- cheese
- pie spice
- 1/2 tsp vanilla
- 4 tsp heavy
- Pinch of salt
- whipping cream

Directions:

1. Turn on Chaffle or chaffle creator. I utilize the Dash Mini, Chaffle Maker.

2. In a little bowl, join all ingredients.

3. Spread the scramble smaller than expected Chaffle creator with 1/4 of the hitter and cook for 3-4

4. minutes.

5. Rehash 3 additional occasions until you have made 4 Maple Syrup

Pumpkin Keto Chaffles

6. Present with sans sugar maple syrup or keto frozen yogurt.

356. Mini Keto Pizza Recipe

Preparation Time: 5minutes
Cooking Time: 10minutes
Servings: 2 Mini Keto Pizzas

Ingredients

- 1/2 cup Shredded
- 1/4 tsp garlic
- Mozzarella cheese
- powder
- 1 tsp almond flour
- 1/4 tsp basil
- 1/2 tsp baking
- 2 tsp low carb pasta
- powder
- sauce
- 1 eggs
- 2 tsp mozzarella
- cheese

Directions:

1. While the Chaffle creator is warming up, in a bowl blend mozzarella cheddar, heating powder, garlic, premise, egg and almond flour.

2. Pour 1/2 the blend into your smaller than normal Chaffle producer.

3. Cook for 3-5 minutes until your pizza Chaffle is totally cooked. In the event that you check it and the Chaffle adheres to the Chaffle producer let it cook for one more moment or two.

4. Next put the rest of the pizza outside layer blend into the Chaffle producer and cook it.

5. When both pizza outsides are cooked, place them on the heating sheet of your toaster stove.

6. Put 1 tsp of low carb pasta sauce over every pizza outside layer.

7. Sprinkle 1 tsp of shredded mozzarella cheddar over everyone.

8. Heat at 350 degrees in the toaster broiler for about 5 minutes, just until the cheddar is softened 76

357. Perfect Pumpkin Spice Chaffles

Preparation Time: 15mins
Cooking Time: 5mins,
Serving: 8

Ingredients

- 4 large eggs
- pint buttermilk
- 2 1/4 tsp baking
- 1 cup canned solid-
- powder
- pack pumpkin
- 2 tsp ground
- 6 tsp unsalted
- cinnamon
- butter
- 1 tsp baking soda
- 2 1/2 cups all-
- 1 tsp ground ginger
- purpose flour
- 1/2 tsp salt
- 1/3 cup packed light
- 1/4 tsp ground
- brown sugar
- cloves

Directions:

1. Preheat a Chaffle iron

2. Beat egg whites in a glass or metallic bowl until delicate pinnacles shape. Lift your mixer or whisk immediately up: the egg whites will form delicate hills in place of a pointy pinnacle.

3. Beat egg yolks, buttermilk, pumpkin, and spread together with a velocity in a massive bowl until smooth; consist of flour, darker sugar, heating powder, cinnamon, making ready pop, ginger, salt, and cloves. Mix the mixture with the whisk simply till you have a easy participant.

4. Overlay the egg whites into the participant just until consolidated.

5. Get geared up cooking surfaces of your Chaffle iron with cooking bathe. Spoon round 2/3 cup

6. participant into the readied iron and cook dinner until caramelized, four to 5 minutes.

358. Banana Chaffles

Preparation Time: 10mins
Cooking Time: 30mins,
Serving: 4

Ingredients

- 1 1/4 Cups All-
- 1 pinch ground
- purpose flour
- nutmeg
- 3 tsp baking powder
- 1 cup milk
- 1/2 tsp salt
- 1 egg
- 2 ripe bananas

Directions:

1. Preheat Chaffle iron. In a huge blending bowl, filter together flour, heating powder, salt, and nutmeg. Mix in milk and eggs until the blend is smooth.

2. Splash preheated Chaffle iron with non-stick cooking shower. Pour two tsp of the Chaffle hitter onto the hot Chaffle iron.

3. Spot two cuts of banana over the hitter and afterward spoon another two tsp of the batter over the banana. Cook until brilliant dark colored.

4. Serve hot.

359. Gingerbread Chaffles With Hot Chocolate Sauce

Preparation Time: 25mins
Cooking Time: 25mins
Serving: 6

Ingredients

- cup light
- ½- tsp ground
- molasses
- cinnamon
- ½- cup butter
- ½- tsp salt
- 1 ½- tsp baking
- cups boiling
- soda
- water
- ½- cup milk
- cup white sugar
- egg
- tsp cornstarch
- cups all-purpose
- ½- cup

- flour
- unsweetened cocoa
- 1 ½- tsp ground
- powder
- ginger
- tsp salt
- tsp vanilla
- tsp butter
- extract

Directions:

1. Remove from warmth and let cool somewhat. Mix in heating pop, milk, and egg.

2. In an enormous bowl, filter together flour, ginger, cinnamon, and salt. Make a well in the middle and pour in the molasses blend.

3. Splash preheated Chaffle iron with non-stick cooking shower. Pour blend into the hot Chaffle iron.

4. Cook until brilliant darker. Serve hot with chocolate sauce. To make chocolate sauce: In a pot, join water, 1 cup sugar, cornstarch, cocoa powder, and 1 tsp salt.

5. Cook over medium warmth, blending continually until blend reaches boiling point.

6. Remove from warmth and include vanilla and 2

7. Tsp spread; mix until smooth.

360. Kate's Light Fluffy Buttermilk And Chocolate Chip Chaffles

Preparation Time: 15mins
Cooking Time: 20mins,
Serving: 10

Ingredients

- 1 ½- cups all-
- ¼- cup heavy
- purpose flour
- cream
- tsp powdered
- egg yolks
- buttermilk
- ¼- cup butter
- 1 ¼- tsp baking
- egg whites
- powder
- cup miniature
- ½- tsp baking soda
- semisweet chocolate
- cup milk
- chips

Directions:

1. In an enormous bowl, blend the flour, powdered buttermilk, heating powder, and preparing pop. In 83

2. a different bowl, whip the cream utilizing an electric blender; mix in milk, egg yolks, and dissolved margarine. Mix the milk blend into the dry ingredients until smooth. In a spotless glass or metal bowl, whip egg whites to solid pinnacles.

3. Overlay the egg whites and chocolate chips into the batter utilizing an elastic spatula or wooden spoon.

4. Preheat a Chaffle iron, and coat with cooking shower. Spoon batter onto the hot iron, and cook until there is never again steam turning out and the Chaffles are light dark-colored.

361. Healthy Multigrain Chia Chaffles

Preparation Time: 15mins
Cooking Time: 20mins
Serving: 8

Ingredients

- 1 3/4 cups almond
- 1 1/4 cups whole
- milk
- wheat flour
- 1/2 cup
- 1/2 cup rolled oats
- unsweetened
- 1/4 cup flax seed
- applesauce
- meal
- 1 egg
- 4 tsp baking powder
- 2 tsp chia seeds
- 2 tsp white sugar
- 1 tsp vanilla extract
- 1/4 tsp salt

Directions:

1. Preheat a Chaffle iron shower within with cooking splash.

2. Whisk almond milk, fruit purée, egg, chia seeds, and vanilla concentrate together in a bowl; let sit until chia seeds begin to thicken the blend, around 2 minutes.

3. Whisk flour, oats, flaxseed supper, preparing powder, sugar, and salt into almond milk blend until the batter is smooth.

4. Scoop 1/2 cup batter into the preheated Chaffle iron and cook until fresh and brilliant, around 5

01. minutes for each Chaffle. Rehash with the rest of the batter.

362. Rich Yogurt Chaffles

Preparation Time: 10mins
Cooking Time: 20mins
Serving: 4

Ingredients

- 3 eggs
- 2 tsp baking powder
- 1 1/2 cups vanilla
- 1 tsp baking soda
- fat-free yogurt
- 1/2 tsp kosher salt
- 1 1/4 cups all-
- 1/2 cup shortening
- purpose flour

Directions:

1. Preheat Chaffle iron. Beat eggs in an enormous blending bowl, at that point include yogurt, flour, heating powder, preparing pop, legitimate salt, and shortening, blending until smooth.

2. Pour batter onto the hot Chaffle iron. Cook until never again steaming, around 5 minutes.

363. Keto Chaffle Taco Shells

Preparation Time: 5minutes
Cooking Time: 20minutes
Servings: 5 Taco Shells

Ingredients

- 1 tsp almond flour
- 1 cup taco blend cheese
- 2 eggs

- 1/4 tsp taco seasoning

Directions:

1. In a bowl blend almond flour, taco mix cheddar, eggs, and taco flavoring. I think that it's most straightforward to blend everything utilizing a fork.

2. Include 1.5 tsp of taco chaffle hitter to the Chaffle creator at once. Cook chaffle batter in the Chaffle creator for 4 minutes.

3. Remove the taco chaffle shell from the Chaffle creator and wrap over the side of a bowl. I utilized my pie container since it was what I had close by however pretty much any bowl will work.

4. Keep making chaffle taco dishes until you are out of the batter. At that point fill your taco shells with taco meat, your preferred ingredients and enjoy!

364. Grain-Free, Low Carb Keto Chaffles

Preparation Time: 5minutes
Cooking Time: 15minutes
Serving: 2

Ingredients

- 1 tsp of almond
- 1 shake of cinnamon
- flour
- 1 tsp baking powder
- 1 egg
- 1 cup mozzarella
- 1 tsp vanilla
- cheese

Directions:

1. In a bowl, combine, egg and vanilla concentrate.

2. Blend in preparing powder, almond flour, and cinnamon.

3. Finally, include the mozzarella cheddar and coat it equitably with the blend.

4. Shower your Chaffle producer with oil and let it heat up to its most noteworthy setting.

5. Cook the Chaffle, minding it at regular intervals until it gets crunchy and brilliant.

6. Making it a muddled procedure. I recommend putting down a silpat tangle for simple cleanup.

7. Take it out cautiously, and top it with spread, and your preferred low-carb syrup.

365. Keto Taco Chaffle

Preparation Time: 10mins
Cooking Time: 8mins
Serving: 4

Ingredients

- Chaffle:
- ¼- tsp salt
- ½- cup cheese
- ½ tsp smoked
- egg
- paprika
- ¼- tsp Italian
- ¼- cup chili powder
- seasoning
- 1/4 cup ground
- tsp chili powder
- cumin
- tsp ground cumin
- tsp garlic powder

178

- ½- tsp garlic
- tsp cocoa powder
- powder
- tsp onion powder
- ½- tsp cocoa
- tsp salt
- powder
- tsp smoked
- ¼- tsp onion
- paprika
- powder

Directions:

1. Cook your floor meat or ground turkey first.

2. Include all of the taco meat seasonings. The cocoa powder is discretionary yet it clearly improves the forms of the various seasonings!

3. While you're making the taco meat, start making the keto chaffles.

4. Spot a huge part of the chaffle blend into the smaller than traditional Chaffle author and cook dinner it for around 3 to 4minutes. Rehash and cook the second one 50% of the blend to make the second chaffle.

5. Add the nice and cozy taco meat to your taco chaffle. Top it with lettuce, tomatoes, cheddar, and serve warm

366. Keto Cornbread Chaffle Recipe

Preparation Time: 10mins
Cooking Time: 8mins
Serving: 3

Ingredients

- 1 egg
- 1 tsp Frank's Red

- 1/2 cup cheddar
- hot sauce
- cheese
- 1/4 tsp corn extract
- 5 slices jalapeno
- pinch salt

Directions:

1. Preheat the more diminutive than everyday Chaffle maker

2. In a bit bowl, whip the egg. Combine the rest of the ingredients and mix it till it is all-round joined.

3. Include a tsp of shredded cheddar to the Chaffle producer for 30 seconds in advance than which comprise the order.

4. This will make a first-rate and smooth outside that is truly extraordinary

5. Add a big part of the combo to the preheated Chaffle producer.

6. Make it for at least three to 4minutes. The longer you make supper it the more energizing it receives.

7. Serve heat and respect it

367. Keto Chaffle Stuffing Recipe

Preparation Time: 10mins
Cooking Time: 35mins
Serving: 4

Ingredients

- Basic Chaffle:
- 1/4 tsp salt
- 1/2 cup cheese,
- 1/4 tsp pepper
- mozzarella
- Stuffing:
- 2 eggs

- 1 small onion
- 1/4 tsp garlic
- 2 celery stalks
- powder
- 4 oz mushrooms
- 1/2 tsp onion
- 4 tbs butter
- powder
- 3 eggs
- 1/2 tsp dried
- poultry seasoning

Directions:

1. To begin with, make your chaffles. Preheat the smaller than normal Chaffle iron. Preheat the stove to 350F

2. In a medium-size bowl, join the chaffle ingredients.

3. Pour a 1/4 of the blend into a smaller than expected Chaffle producer and cook each chaffle for around 4 minutes each.

4. In a little griddle, saute the onion, celery, and mushrooms until they are delicate.

5. In a different bowl, destroy the chaffles into little pieces, include the sauteed veggies and 3 eggs.

6. Blend until the ingredients are completely joined.

7. Add the stuffing blend to a little goulash dish and prepare it at 350 degrees for around 30 to 40

8. minutes. Serve warm and enjoy

368. Chicken Zinger Chaffle

Preparation Time: 15 min
Cooking Time: 15 min
Servings: 2

Ingredients

- 1 chicken breast, cut into 2 pieces
- 1/2 cup coconut flour
- 1/4 cup finely grated Parmesan
- 1 tsp. paprika
- 1/2 tsp. garlic powder
- 1/2 tsp. onion powder
- 1 tsp. salt& pepper
- 1 egg beaten
- Avocado oil for frying
- Lettuce leaves
- BBQ sauce
- Chaffle Ingredients
- 4 oz. cheese
- 2 whole eggs
- 2 oz. almond flour
- 1/4 cup almond flour
- 1 tsp baking powder

Directions

1. Mix together chaffle ingredients in a bowl.

2. Pour the chaffle batter in preheated greased square chaffle maker.

3. Cook chaffles for about 2-3 minutes until cooked through.

4. Make 4 square chaffles from this batter.

5. Meanwhile mix together coconut flour, parmesan, paprika, garlic powder, onion powder salt and pepper in a bowl.

6. Dip chicken first in coconut flour mixture then in beaten egg.

7. Heat avocado oil in a skillet and cook chicken from both sides. until lightly brown and cooked

8. Set chicken zinger between two chaffles with lettuce and BBQ sauce.

9. Enjoy!

369. Chaffle & Chicken Lunch Plate

Preparation Time: 5 min
Cooking Time: 15 min
Servings: 1

Ingredients

- 1 large egg
- 1/2 cup jack cheese, shredded
- 1 pinch salt
- For Serving
- 1 chicken leg
- salt
- pepper
- 1 tsp. garlic, minced
- 1 egg
- I tsp avocado oil

Directions

1. Heat your square waffle maker and grease with cooking spray.

2. Pour Chaffle batter intothe skillet and cook for about 2-3 minutes.

3. Meanwhile,heat oil in a pan, over medium heat.

4. Once the oil is hot, add chicken thigh and garlicthen, cook for about 4-5 minutes. Flip and cook for another 3-4 minutes.

5. Season with salt and pepper and give them a good mix.

6. Transfer cooked thigh to plate.

7. Fry the egg in the same pan for about 1-2 minutes according to your choice.

8. Once chaffles are cooked, serve with fried egg and chicken thigh.

9. Enjoy!

370. Grill Pork Chaffle Sandwich

Preparation Time: 5 min
Cooking Time: 15 min
Servings: 2

Ingredients

- 1/2 cup mozzarella, shredded
- 1 egg
- I pinch garlic powder
- Pork Patty
- 1/2 cup pork, minced
- 1 tbsp. green onion, diced
- 1/2 tsp Italian seasoning
- Lettuce leaves

Directions

1. Preheat the square waffle maker and grease with

2. Mix together egg, cheese and garlic powder in a small mixing bowl.

3. Pour batter in a preheated waffle maker and close the lid.

4. Make 2 chaffles from thisbatter.

5. Cook chaffles for about 2-3 minutes until cooked through.

6. Meanwhile, mix together pork patty ingredients in a bowl and make 1 large patty.

7. Grill pork patty in a preheated grill for about 3-4 minutes per side until cooked through.

8. Arrange pork patty between two chaffles with lettuce leaves. Cut sandwich to make a triangular sandwich.

9. Enjoy!

371. Crunchy Fish And Chaffle Bites

Preparation Time: 15 min
Cooking Time: 15 min
Servings: 4

Ingredients

- 1 lb. cod fillets, sliced into 4 slice
- 1 tsp. sea salt
- 1 tsp. garlic powder
- 1 egg, whisked
- 1 cup almond flour
- 2 tbsp. avocado oil
- Chaffle Ingredients
- 2 eggs
- 1/2 cup cheddar cheese
- 2 tbsps. almond flour
- ½ tsp. Italian seasoning

Directions

1. Mix together chaffle ingredients in a bowl and make 4 square
2. Put the chaffles in a preheated chaffle maker.
3. Mix together the salt, pepper, and garlic powder in a mixing bowl. Toss the cod cubes in this mixture and let sit for 10 minutes.
4. Then dip each cod slice into the egg mixture and then into the almond flour.
5. Heat oil in skillet and fish cubes for about 2-3 minutes, until cooked and browned
6. Serve on chaffles and enjoy!

372. Double Chicken Chaffles

Preparation Time: 5 min
Cooking Time: 5 min
Servings: 2

Ingredients

- 1/2 Cup Boil Shredded Chicken
- 1/4 Cup Cheddar Cheese
- 1/8 Cup Parmesan Cheese
- 1 Egg
- 1 Tsp. Italian Seasoning
- 1/8 Tsp. Garlic Powder
- 1 Tsp. Cream Cheese

Directions

1. Preheat the Belgian waffle maker.
2. Mix together in chaffle ingredients in a bowl and mix together.
3. Sprinkle 1 tbsp. of cheese in a waffle maker and pour in chaffle batter.
4. Pour 1 tbsp. of cheese over batter and close the lid.
5. Cook chaffles for about 4 to 5 minutes.
6. Serve with a chicken zinger and enjoy the double chicken flavor.

373. Chicken Bites With Chaffles

Preparation Time: 5 Min
Cooking Time: 10 min
Servings: 2

Ingredients

- 1 chicken breastscut into 2 x2 inch chunks
- 1 egg, whisked
- 1/4 cup almond flour
- 2 tbsps. onion powder
- 2 tbsps. garlic powder
- 1 tsp. dried oregano
- 1 tsp. paprika powder
- 1 tsp. salt
- 1/2 tsp. black pepper

- 2 tbsps. avocado oil

Directions

1. Add all the dry ingredients together into a large bowl. Mix well.

2. Place the eggs into a separate bowl.

3. Dip each chicken piece into the egg and then into the dry ingredients.

4. Heat oil in 10-inch skillet, add oil.

5. Once avocado oil is hot, place the coated chicken nuggets onto a skillet and cook for 6-8 minutes until cooked and golden brown.

6. Serve with chaffles and raspberries.

7. Enjoy!

374. Cauliflower Chaffles And Tomatoes

Preparation Time: 5 min
Cooking Time: 15 min
Servings: 2

Ingredients

- 1/2 cup cauliflower
- 1/4 tsp. garlic powder
- 1/4 tsp. black pepper
- 1/4 tsp. Salt
- 1/2 cup shredded cheddar cheese
- 1 egg
- For Topping
- 1 lettuce leave
- 1 tomato sliced
- 4 oz. cauliflower steamed, mashed
- 1 tsp sesame seeds

Directions

1. Add all chaffle ingredients into a blender and mix well.

2. Sprinkle 1/8 shredded cheese on the waffle maker and pour cauliflower mixture in a preheated waffle maker and sprinkle the rest of the cheese over it.

3. Cook chaffles for about 4-5 minutes until cooked

4. For serving, lay lettuce leaves over chaffle top with steamed cauliflower and tomato.

5. Drizzle sesame seeds on top.

6. Enjoy!

375. Chaffle With Cheese & Bacon

Preparation Time: 15 min
Cooking Time: 15 min
Servings: 2

Ingredients

- 1 egg
- 1/2 cup cheddar cheese, shredded
- 1 tbsp. parmesan cheese
- 3/4 tsp coconut flour
- 1/4 tsp baking powder
- 1/8 tsp Italian Seasoning
- pinch of salt
- 1/4 tsp garlic powder
- For Topping
- 1 bacon sliced, cooked and chopped
- 1/2 cup mozzarella cheese, shredded
- 1/4 tsp parsley, chopped

Directions

1. Preheat oven to 400 degrees.

2. Switch on your mini waffle maker and grease with cooking spray.

3. Mix together chaffle ingredients in a mixing bowl until combined.

4. Spoon half of the batter in the center of the waffle maker and close the lid. Cook chaffles for about 3-4 minutes until cooked.

5. Carefully remove chaffles from the maker.

6. Arrange chaffles in a greased baking tray.

7. Top with mozzarella cheese, chopped bacon and parsley.

8. And bake in the oven for 4 -5 minutes.

9. Once the cheese is melted, remove from the oven.

10. Serve and enjoy!

376. Chaffle Mini Sandwich

Preparation Time: 5 min
Cooking Time: 10 min
Servings: 2

Ingredients

- 1 large egg
- 1/8 cup almond flour
- 1/2 tsp. garlic powder
- 3/4 tsp. baking powder
- 1/2 cup shredded cheese
- Sandwich Filling
- 2 slices deli ham
- 2 slices tomatoes
- 1 slice cheddar cheese

Directions

1. Grease your square waffle maker and preheat it on medium heat.

2. Mix together chaffle ingredients in a mixing bowl until well combined.

3. Pour batter intoa square waffle and make two chaffles.

4. Once chaffles are cooked, remove from the maker.

5. For a sandwich, arrange deli ham, tomato slice and cheddar cheese between two chaffles.

6. Cut sandwich from the center.

7. Serve and enjoy!

377. Chaffles With Topping

Preparation Time: 5 min
Cooking Time: 10 min
Servings: 3
Ingredients

- 1 large egg
- 1 tbsp. almond flour
- 1 tbsp. full-fat Greek yogurt
- 1/8 tsp baking powder
- 1/4 cup shredded Swiss cheese
- Topping
- 4oz. grillprawns
- 4 oz. steamed cauliflower mash
- 1/2 zucchini sliced
- 3 lettuce leaves
- 1 tomato, sliced
- 1 tbsp. flax seeds

Directions

1. Make 3 chaffles with the given chaffles ingredients.

2. For serving, arrange lettuce leaves on each chaffle.

3. Top with zucchini slice, grill prawns, cauliflower mash and a tomato slice.

4. Drizzle flax seeds on top.

5. Serve and enjoy!

378. Grill Beefsteak And Chaffle

Preparation Time: 5 min
Cooking Time: 10 min
Servings: 1

Ingredients

- 1 beefsteak rib eye
- 1 tsp salt
- 1 tsp pepper
- 1 tbsp. lime juice
- 1 tsp garlic

Directions

1. Prepare your grill for direct heat.
2. Mix together all spices and rub over beefsteak evenly.
3. Place the beef on the grill rack over medium heat.
4. Cover and cook steak for about6 to 8 minutes. Flip and cook for another 4-5 minutes until cooked through.
5. Serve with keto simple chaffle and enjoy!

379. Barbecue Chaffle

Preparation Time: 5 minutes
Cooking Time: 8 minutes
Servings: 2

Ingredients:

- 1 egg, beaten
- ½ cup cheddar cheese, shredded
- ½ teaspoon barbecue sauce
- ¼ teaspoon baking powder

Directions:

1. Plug in your waffle maker to preheat.
2. Mix all the ingredients in a bowl.
3. Pour half of the mixture to your waffle maker.

4. Cover and cook for 4 minutes.
5. Repeat the same steps for the next barbecue chaffle.

380. Turkey Chaffle Burger

Preparation Time: 10 minutes
Cooking Time: 10 minutes
Servings: 2

Ingredients:

- 2 cups ground turkey
- Salt and pepper to taste
- 1 tablespoon olive oil
- 4 garlic chaffles
- 1 cup Romaine lettuce, chopped
- 1 tomato, sliced
- Mayonnaise
- Ketchup

Directions:

1. Combine ground turkey, salt and pepper.
2. Form 2 thick burger patties.
3. Add the olive oil to a pan over medium heat.
4. Cook the turkey burger until fully cooked on both sides.
5. Spread mayo on the chaffle.
6. Top with the turkey burger, lettuce and tomato.
7. Squirt ketchup on top before topping with another chaffle.

381. Savory Beef Chaffle

Preparation Time: 10 minutes
Cooking Time: 15 minutes
Servings: 2

Ingredients:

- 1 teaspoon olive oil
- 2 cups ground beef
- Garlic salt to taste
- 1 red bell pepper, sliced into strips
- 1 green bell pepper, sliced into strips
- 1 onion, minced
- 1 bay leaf
- 2 garlic chaffles
- Butter

Directions:

1. Put your pan over medium heat.
2. Add the olive oil and cook ground beef until brown.
3. Season with garlic salt and add bay leaf.
4. Drain the fat, transfer to a plate and set aside.
5. Discard the bay leaf.
6. In the same pan, cook the onion and bell peppers for 2 minutes.
7. Put the beef back to the pan.
8. Heat for 1 minute.
9. Spread butter on top of the chaffle.
10. Add the ground beef and veggies.
11. Roll or fold the chaffle.

382. Spicy Shrimp and Chaffles

Preparation Time: 15 minutes
Cooking Time: 31 minutes
Servings: 4

Ingredients:

- For the shrimp:
- 1 tbsp olive oil
- 1 lb jumbo shrimp, peeled and deveined

- 1 tbsp Creole seasoning
- Salt to taste
- 2 tbsp hot sauce
- 3 tbsp butter
- 2 tbsp chopped fresh scallions to garnish
- For the chaffles:
- 2 eggs, beaten
- 1 cup finely grated Monterey Jack cheese

Directions:

1. For the shrimp:
2. Heat the olive oil in a medium skillet over medium heat.
3. Season the shrimp with the Creole seasoning and salt. Cook in the oil until pink and opaque on both sides, 2 minutes.
4. Pour in the hot sauce and butter. Mix well until the shrimp is adequately coated in the sauce, 1 minute.
5. Turn the heat off and set aside.
6. For the chaffles:
7. Preheat the waffle iron.
8. In a medium bowl, mix the eggs and Monterey Jack cheese.
9. Open the iron and add a quarter of the mixture. Close and cook until crispy, 7 minutes.
10. Transfer the chaffle to a plate and make 3 more chaffles in the same manner.
11. Cut the chaffles into quarters and place on a plate.
12. Top with the shrimp and garnish with the scallions.
13. Serve warm.

383. Chicken Jalapeño Chaffles

Preparation Time: 15 minutes
Cooking Time: 14 minutes
Servings: 2

Ingredients:

- 1/8 cup finely grated Parmesan cheese
- ¼ cup finely grated cheddar cheese
- 1 egg, beaten
- ½ cup cooked chicken breasts, diced
- 1 small jalapeño pepper, deseeded and minced
- 1/8 tsp garlic powder
- 1/8 tsp onion powder
- 1 tsp cream cheese, softened

Directions:

1. Preheat the waffle iron.
2. In a medium bowl, mix all the ingredients until adequately combined.
3. Open the iron and add half of the mixture. Close and cook until crispy, 7 minutes.
4. Transfer the chaffle to a plate and make a second chaffle in the same manner.
5. Allow cooling and serve afterward.

384. Chicken and Chaffle Nachos

Preparation Time: 15 minutes
Cooking Time: 33 minutes
Servings: 4

Ingredients:

- For the chaffles:
- 2 eggs, beaten
- 1 cup finely grated Mexican cheese blend

- For the chicken-cheese topping:
- 2 tbsp butter
- 1 tbsp almond flour
- ¼ cup unsweetened almond milk
- 1 cup finely grated cheddar cheese + more to garnish
- 3 bacon slices, cooked and chopped
- 2 cups cooked and diced chicken breasts
- 2 tbsp hot sauce
- 2 tbsp chopped fresh scallions

Directions:

1. For the chaffles:
2. Preheat the waffle iron.
3. In a medium bowl, mix the eggs and Mexican cheese blend.
4. Open the iron and add a quarter of the mixture. Close and cook until crispy, 7 minutes.
5. Transfer the chaffle to a plate and make 3 more chaffles in the same manner.
6. Place the chaffles on serving plates and set aside for serving.
7. For the chicken-cheese topping:
8. Melt the butter in a large skillet and mix in the almond flour until brown, 1 minute.
9. Pour the almond milk and whisk until well combined. Simmer until thickened, 2 minutes.
10. Stir in the cheese to melt, 2 minutes and then mix in the bacon, chicken, and hot sauce.
11. Spoon the mixture onto the chaffles and top with some more cheddar cheese.
12. Garnish with the scallions and serve

immediately.

385. Buffalo Hummus Beef Chaffles

Preparation Time: 15 minutes
Cooking Time: 32 minutes
Servings: 4

Ingredients:

- 2 eggs
- 1 cup + ¼ cup finely grated cheddar cheese, divided
- 2 chopped fresh scallions
- Salt and freshly ground black pepper to taste
- 2 chicken breasts, cooked and diced
- ¼ cup buffalo sauce
- 3 tbsp low-carb hummus
- 2 celery stalks, chopped
- ¼ cup crumbled blue cheese for topping

Directions:

1. Preheat the waffle iron.
2. In a medium bowl, mix the eggs, 1 cup of the cheddar cheese, scallions, salt, and black pepper,
3. Open the iron and add a quarter of the mixture. Close and cook until crispy, 7 minutes.
4. Transfer the chaffle to a plate and make 3 more chaffles in the same manner.
5. Preheat the oven to 400 F and line a baking sheet with parchment paper. Set aside.
6. Cut the chaffles into quarters and arrange on the baking sheet.
7. In a medium bowl, mix the chicken with the buffalo sauce, hummus, and celery.

8. Spoon the chicken mixture onto each quarter of chaffles and top with the remaining cheddar cheese.
9. Place the baking sheet in the oven and bake until the cheese melts, 4 minutes.
10. Remove from the oven and top with the blue cheese.
11. Serve afterward.

386. Pork Rind Chaffle

Preparation time: 10 minutes
Cooking time: 20 minutes
Servings: 4 medium chaffles

Ingredients:

- 1 1/3 cup / 150 grams shredded mozzarella cheese
- 4 eggs, at room temperature
- 2 cups / 475 grams crushed pork rinds
- Sour cream for topping

Directions:

1. Take a non-stick waffle iron, plug it in, select the medium or medium-high heat setting and let it preheat until ready to use; it could also be indicated with an indicator light changing its color.
2. Meanwhile, prepare the batter, and for this, place pork rind in a food processor and process for 1 minute until mixture resembles grains.
3. Take a large bowl, crack eggs in it, add pork rinds and cheese, and mix with a hand whisk until smooth.
4. Use a ladle to pour one-fourth of the prepared batter into the heated waffle iron in a spiral direction, starting from the edges, then shut the lid and cook for 5 minutes or more until solid and

nicely browned; the cooked waffle will look like a cake.

5. When done, transfer chaffles to a plate with a silicone spatula and repeat with the remaining batter.

6. Let chaffles stand for some time until crispy, top with a dollop of sour cream and serve.

387. Cheesy Chicken and Ham Chaffle

Preparation time: 5 minutes
Cooking time: 12 minutes
Servings: 4 mini chaffles

Ingredients:

- 4 tablespoons chopped ham
- 1/4 cup / 60 grams diced chicken, cooked
- 1/4 cup / 30 grams shredded Swiss cheese
- 1 egg, at room temperature
- 1/4 cup / 30 grams shredded mozzarella cheese

Directions:

1. Take a non-stick mini waffle iron, plug it in, select the medium or medium-high heat setting and let it preheat until ready to use; it could also be indicated with an indicator light changing its color.

2. Meanwhile, prepare the batter and for this, take a large bowl, crack eggs in it, beat with a hand whisk, then add remaining ingredients and whisk until incorporated.

3. Use a ladle to pour one-fourth of the prepared batter into the heated waffle iron in a spiral direction, starting from the edges, then shut the lid and cook for 4 minutes or more until solid and nicely browned; the cooked waffle

will look like a cake.

4. When done, transfer chaffles to a plate with a silicone spatula and repeat with the remaining batter.

5. Let chaffles stand for some time until crispy and serve straight away.

388. Cloud Bread Cheddar Chaffle

Preparation time: 10 minutes
Cooking time: 20 minutes
Servings: 4

Ingredients:

- ¼ cup / 60 grams whey protein powder
- ¼ teaspoon salt
- ½ teaspoon baking powder
- ¼ cup / 60 grams sour cream
- ½ cup / 55 shredded cheddar cheese
- 3 eggs, at room temperature
- Crispy bacon for topping
- Chopped chives for topping

Directions:

1. Take a non-stick waffle iron, plug it in, select the medium or medium-high heat setting and let it preheat until ready to use; it could also be indicated with an indicator light changing its color.

2. Meanwhile, prepare the batter and for this, take a large bowl, crack eggs in it, add remaining ingredients except for the toppings and then stir with an electric mixer until smooth.

3. Use a ladle to pour one-fourth of the prepared batter into the heated waffle iron in a spiral direction, starting from the edges, then shut the lid and cook for 5 minutes or more until solid and nicely browned; the cooked waffle will look like a cake.

4. When done, transfer chaffles to a plate with a silicone spatula and repeat with the remaining batter.

5. Let chaffles stand for some time until crispy, then top with bacon, sprinkle with chives, and serve straight away.

389. Corn Bread Chaffle

Preparation time: 10 minutes
Cooking time: 20 minutes
Servings: 4 medium chaffles

Ingredients:

- 3 cups / 290 grams ground almonds, blanched
- 2 teaspoons baking soda
- 8 tablespoons hemp seeds
- 1 teaspoon baking powder
- 1 teaspoon of sea salt
- 4 tablespoons avocado oil
- 8 tablespoons coconut milk, unsweetened
- 4 eggs, at room temperature

Directions:

1. Take a non-stick waffle iron, plug it in, select the medium or medium-high heat setting and let it preheat until ready to use; it could also be indicated with an indicator light changing its color.

2. Meanwhile, prepare the batter and for this, take a large bowl, add almonds and seeds in it and then stir in salt, baking powder, and soda until combined.

3. Take a separate bowl, crack eggs in it, add oil, pour in milk, stir with a hand whisk until frothy, and then stir this mixture with a spoon into the almond mixture until incorporated.

4. Use a ladle to pour one-fourth of the prepared batter into the heated waffle iron in a spiral direction, starting from the edges, then shut the lid and cook for 5 minutes or more until solid and nicely browned; the cooked waffle will look like a cake.

5. When done, transfer chaffles to a plate with a silicone spatula and repeat with the remaining batter.

6. Let chaffles stand for some time until crispy and serve straight away.

390. Brie, Basil and Tomato Chaffle

Preparation time: 10 minutes
Cooking time: 24 minutes
Servings: 4 mini chaffles

Ingredients:

- 4 cherry tomatoes, diced
- 1 teaspoon dried basil
- 1 cup / 235 grams Brie cheese cubes, softened
- 2 eggs, at room temperature

Directions:

1. Take a non-stick mini waffle iron, plug it in, select the medium or medium-high heat setting and let it preheat until ready to use; it could also be indicated with an indicator light changing its color.

2. Meanwhile, prepare the batter and for this, take a large bowl, crack eggs in it, add cheese, tomatoes, and basil and mix with a hand whisk until combined.

3. Use a ladle to pour one-fourth of the prepared batter into the heated waffle iron in a spiral direction, starting from the edges, then shut the lid and cook for 4 to 6 minutes until solid and nicely browned; the cooked waffle will look like a cake.

4. When done, transfer chaffles to a plate with a silicone spatula and repeat with the remaining batter.

5. Let chaffles stand for some time until crispy and serve straight away.

391. Broccoli Chaffle

Preparation time: 10 minutes
Cooking time: 15 minutes
Servings: 3 medium chaffles

Ingredients:

- 1 cup / 175 grams broccoli florets
- 2 eggs, at room temperature
- 6 tablespoons grated parmesan cheese
- 1 cup / 115 grams shredded cheddar cheese

Directions:

1. Take a non-stick waffle iron, plug it in, select the medium or medium-high heat setting and let it preheat until ready to use; it could also be indicated with an indicator light changing its color.

2. Meanwhile, prepare the batter, and for this, place broccoli florets in a blender and pulse for 1 to 2 minutes until florets resemble rice.

3. Tip the broccoli in a medium bowl, add remaining ingredients and then stir with a hand whisk until combined.

4. Use a ladle to pour one-third of the prepared batter into the heated waffle iron in a spiral direction, starting from the edges, then shut the lid and cook for 5 minutes or more until solid and nicely browned; the cooked waffle will look like a cake.

5. When done, transfer chaffles to a plate with a silicone spatula and repeat

with the remaining batter.

01. Let chaffles stand for some time until crispy and serve straight away.

392. Cheesy Spinach Chaffle

Preparation time: 10 minutes
Cooking time: 20 minutes
Servings: 4 large chaffles

Ingredients:

- 1 cup / 225 grams frozen baby spinach, thawed
- ½ teaspoon ground black pepper
- ½ teaspoon salt
- ½ teaspoon cumin
- 1 cup / 115 grams grated cheddar cheese
- 8 eggs, at room temperature
- For the Avocado Sauce:
- 1 medium avocado, pitted, diced
- ¼ teaspoon ground black pepper
- 1/3 teaspoon salt
- 2 limes, juiced
- 2 tablespoons coconut milk, unsweetened

Directions:

1. Take a non-stick waffle iron, plug it in, select the medium or medium-high heat setting and let it preheat until ready to use; it could also be indicated with an indicator light changing its color.

2. Meanwhile, prepare the batter for the chaffles, and for this, squeeze moisture from the spinach in a fine sieve as much as possible and then chop it.

3. Take a large bowl, add spinach in it along with cheese, cumin, black

pepper, salt and eggs, and stir with a hand whisk until smooth.

4. Use a ladle to pour one-fourth of the prepared batter into the heated waffle iron in a spiral direction, starting from the edges, then shut the lid and cook for 5 minutes or more until solid and nicely browned; the cooked waffle will look like a cake.

5. When done, transfer chaffles to a plate with a silicone spatula and repeat with the remaining batter.

6. In the meantime, prepare the sauce, and for this, place diced avocado in a blender along with remaining ingredients and process for 1 minute until smooth.

7. Let chaffles stand for some time until crispy, then drizzle with prepared avocado sauce and serve straight away.

393 Chaffle Bread Sticks

Preparation time: 10 minutes
Cooking time: 13 minutes
Servings: 2 medium chaffles

Ingredients:

- For Chaffles:
- 2 tablespoons almond flour
- 1/2 teaspoon dried oregano
- 1/2 teaspoon garlic powder
- 1/2 teaspoon salt
- 1/2 cup / 60 grams grated mozzarella cheese
- 1 egg, at room temperature
- For Topping:
- 1/4 cup / 30 grams grated mozzarella cheese
- 1/2 teaspoon garlic powder

- 2 tablespoons coconut butter, unsalted, softened

Directions:

1. Take a non-stick waffle iron, plug it in, select the medium or medium-high heat setting and let it preheat until ready to use; it could also be indicated with an indicator light changing its color.

2. Meanwhile, prepare the batter and for this, take a large bowl, crack the egg in it, add flour, oregano, garlic powder, salt, and mozzarella cheese and mix with an electric mixer until incorporated.

3. Use a ladle to pour half of the prepared batter into the heated waffle iron in a spiral direction, starting from the edges, then shut the lid and cook for 5 minutes or more until solid and nicely browned; the cooked waffle will look like a cake.

4. When done, transfer chaffles to a plate with a silicone spatula and repeat with the remaining batter.

5. Meanwhile, prepare the topping and for this, take a small bowl, add garlic and butter in it and stir well until combined.

6. Let chaffles stand for some time until crispy, then arrange them on a heatproof tray, and drizzle the topping on top.

7. Preheat the grill over medium-high heat, and when hot, place the tray containing chaffle sticks and grill for 3 minutes until cheese has melted.

8. Serve straight away.

394. Spinach Artichoke Chaffle with Bacon

Preparation time: 5 mins

Cooking time: 8 mins
Servings: 2

Ingredients:

- 4 slices of bacon
- ½ cup chopped spinach
- 1/3 cup marinated artichoke (chopped)
- 1 egg
- ¼ tsp garlic powder
- ¼ tsp smoked paprika
- 2 tbsp cream cheese (softened)
- 1/3 cup shredded mozzarella

Directions:

1. Heat up a frying pan and add the bacon slices. Sear until both sides of the bacon slices are browned. Use a slotted spoon to transfer the bacon to a paper towel line plate to drain.

2. Once the bacon slices are cool, chop them into bits and set aside.

3. Plug the waffle maker to preheat it and spray it with a non-stick cooking spray.

4. In a mixing bowl, combine mozzarella, garlic, paprika, cream cheese and egg. Mix until the ingredients are well combined.

5. Add the spinach, artichoke and bacon bit. Mix until they are well incorporated.

6. Pour an appropriate amount of the batter into the waffle maker and spread the batter to the edges to cover all the holes on the waffle maker.

7. Close the waffle maker and cook 4 minutes or more, according to your waffle maker's settings.

8. After the cooking cycle, use a silicone or plastic utensil to remove the chaffle from the waffle maker.

9. Repeat step 6 to 8 until you have cooked all the batter into chaffles.

10. Serve and top with sour cream as desired.

395. Lobster Chaffle

Preparation time: 5 mins
Cooking time: 8 mins
Servings: 2

Ingredients:

- 1 egg (beaten)
- ½ cup shredded mozzarella cheese
- ¼ tsp garlic powder
- ¼ tsp onion powder
- 1/8 tsp Italian seasoning
- Lobster Filling:
- ½ cup lobster tails (defrosted)
- 1 tbsp mayonnaise
- 1 tsp dried basil
- 1 tsp lemon juice
- 1 tbsp chopped green onion

Directions:

1. Plug the waffle maker to preheat it and spray it with a non-stick cooking spray.

2. In a mixing bowl, combine the mozzarella, Italian seasoning, garlic and onion powder. Add the egg and mix until the ingredients are well combined.

3. Pour an appropriate amount of the batter into the waffle maker and

spread out the batter to cover all the holes on the waffle maker.

4. Close the waffle maker and cook for about 4 minutes or according to your waffle maker's settings.

5. After the cooking cycle, use a plastic or silicone utensil to remove and transfer the chaffle to a wire rack to cool.

6. Repeat step 3 to 5 until you have cooked all the batter into chaffles.

7. For the filling, put the lobster tail in a mixing bowl and add the mayonnaise, basil and lemon juice. Toss until the ingredients are well combine.

8. Fill the chaffles with the lobster mixture and garnish with chopped green onion.

9. Serve and enjoy.

396. Savory Pork Rind Chaffle

Preparation time: 5 mins
Cooking time: 10 minutes
Servings: 2

Ingredients:

- ¼ tsp paprika
- ¼ tsp oregano
- ¼ tsp garlic powder
- 1/8 tsp ground black pepper or to taste
- ½ onion (finely chopped)
- ½ cup pork rind (crushed)
- ½ cup mozzarella cheese
- 1 large egg (beaten)

Directions:

1. Plug the waffle maker to preheat it and spray I with a non-stick cooking spray.

2. In a mixing bowl, combine the crushed pork rind, cheese, onion, paprika, garlic powder and pepper. Add the egg and mix until the ingredients are well combined.

3. Pour an appropriate amount of the batter into the waffle maker and spread out the batter to cover all the holes on the waffle maker.

4. Close the waffle maker and cook for about 5 minutes or according to your waffle maker's settings.

5. After the cooking cycle, use a plastic or silicone utensil to remove the chaffle from the waffle maker.

6. Repeat step 3 to 5 until you have cooked all the batter into chaffles.

7. Serve and top with sour cream as desired.

397.. Shrimp Avocado Chaffle Sandwich

Preparation time: 10 mins
Cooking time: 32 mins
Servings: 4

Ingredients:

- 2 cups shredded mozzarella cheese
- 4 large eggs
- ½ tsp curry powder
- ½ tsp oregano
- Shrimp Sandwich Filling:
- 1-pound raw shrimp (peeled and deveined)
- 1 large avocado (diced)
- 4 slices cooked bacon
- 2 tbsp sour cream
- ½ tsp paprika
- 1 tsp Cajun seasoning

- 1 tbsp olive oil
- ¼ cup onion (finely chopped)
- 1 red bell pepper (diced)

Directions:

1. Plug the waffle maker to preheat it and spray it with a non-stick cooking spray.
2. Break the eggs into a mixing bowl and beat. Add the cheese, oregano and curry. Mix until the ingredients are well combined.
3. Pour an appropriate amount of the batter into the waffle maker and spread out the batter to the edges to cover all the holes on the waffle maker. This should make 8 mini waffles.
4. Close the waffle maker and cook for about 4 minutes or according to your waffle maker's settings.
5. After the cooking cycle, use a silicone or plastic utensil to remove the chaffle from the waffle maker.
6. Repeat step 3 to 5 until you have cooked all the batter into chaffles.
7. Heat up the olive oil in a large skillet over medium to high heat.
8. Add the shrimp and cook until the shrimp is pink and tender.
9. Remove the skillet from heat and use a slotted spoon to transfer the shrimp to a paper towel lined plate to drain for a few minutes.
10. Put the shrimp in a mixing bowl. Add paprika and Cajun seasoning. Toss until the shrimps are all coated with seasoning.
11. To assemble the sandwich, place one chaffle on a flat surface and spread some sour cream over it. Layer some shrimp, onion, avocado, diced pepper and one slice of bacon over it. Cover

with another chaffle.

12. Repeat step 10 until you have assembled all the ingredients into sandwiches.
13. Serve and enjoy.

398. Keto Protein Chaffle

Preparation time: 5 mins
Cooking time: 8 mins
Servings: 1

Ingredients:

- 1 egg (beaten)
- ½ cup whey protein powder
- A pinch of salt
- 1 tsp baking powder
- 3 tbsp sour cream
- ½ tsp vanilla extract
- Topping:
- 2 tbsp heavy cream
- 1 tbsp granulated swerve

Directions:

1. Plug the waffle maker to preheat it and spray it with a non-stick cooking spray.
2. In a mixing bowl, whisk together the egg, vanilla and sour cream.
3. In another mixing bowl, combine the protein powder, baking powder and salt.
4. Pour the flour mixture into the egg mixture and mix until the ingredients are well combined and you form a smooth batter.
5. Pour an appropriate amount of the batter into the waffle maker and spread the batter to the edges to cover all the holes on the waffle maker.

6. Close the waffle maker and cook for about 4 minutes or according to your waffle maker's settings.

7. After the cooking cycle, use a plastic or silicone utensil to remove the chaffle from the waffle iron.

8. Repeat step 4 to 6 until you have cooked all the batter into chaffles.

9. For the topping, whisk together the cream and swerve in a mixing bowl until smooth and fluffy.

10. Top the chaffles with the cream and enjoy.

399. Cauliflower Hash Brown Chaffle

Preparation time: 10 mins
Cooking time: 8 mins
Servings: 2

Ingredients:

- 1 egg
- ½ cup cauliflower rice
- ¼ tsp onion powder
- ¼ tsp salt
- ½ tsp garlic powder
- 4 tbsp shredded cheddar cheese
- 1 green onion (chopped)

Directions:

1. Put the cauliflower rice in a microwave safe dish and cover the dish. Place the dish in the microwave and microwave for 3 minutes.

2. Remove the dish from the microwave and stir. Return it to the microwave and steam for about 1 minute or until tender.

3. Let the steamed cauliflower cool for a few minutes. Wrap the steamed cauliflower in a clean towel and

squeeze it to remove excess water.

4. Plug the waffle maker to preheat it and spray it with a non-stick cooking spray.

5. In a mixing bowl, combine the cauliflower, green onion, onion powder, cheese, salt, garlic and salt. Add the egg and mix until the ingredients are well combined.

6. Fill your waffle maker with an appropriate amount of the batter and spread out the batter to cover all the holes on the waffle maker.

7. Close the waffle maker and cook until the chaffle is browned. This will take about 4 minutes or more depending on your waffle maker.

8. After the cooking cycle, use a plastic or silicone utensil to remove the chaffle from the waffle maker.

9. Repeat step 6 to 8 until you have cooked all the batter into waffles.

10. Serve the hash brown chaffles and top with your desired topping.

400. Shirataki Rice Chaffle

Preparation time: 5 mins
Cooking time: 20 mins
Servings: 4

Ingredients:

- 2 tbsp almond flour
- ½ tsp oregano
- 1 bag of shirataki rice
- 1 tsp baking powder
- 1 cup shredded cheddar cheese
- 2 eggs (beaten)

Directions:

1. Rinse the shirataki rice with warm water for about 30 seconds and rinse it.

2. Plug the waffle maker to preheat it and spray it with a non-stick cooking spray.

3. In a mixing bowl, combine the rinsed rice, almond flour, baking powder, oregano and shredded cheese. Add the eggs and mix until the ingredients are well combined.

4. Fill the waffle maker with an appropriate amount of the batter and spread out the batter to the edges to cover all the holes on the waffle maker.

5. Close the waffle make and cook for about 5 minutes or according to you waffle maker's settings.

6. After the cooking cycle, use a silicone or plastic utensil to remove the chaffles from the waffle maker.

7. Repeat step 4 to 6 until you have cooked all the batter into chaffles.

8. Serve and enjoy.

401. Savory Chaffle Stick

Preparation time: 10 mins
Cooking time: 25 mins
Servings: 16

Ingredients:

- 6 eggs
- 2 cups shredded mozzarella cheese
- A pinch of salt
- ½ tsp ground black pepper or to taste
- ½ tsp baking powder
- 4 tbsp coconut flour
- 1 tsp onion powder
- 1 tsp garlic powder
- 1 tsp oregano
- ¼ tsp Italian seasoning
- 1 tbsp olive oil

- 1 tbsp melted butter

Directions:

1. Plug the waffle maker to preheat it and spray it with a non-stick cooking spray.

2. Break 4 of the eggs into a mixing bowl and beat. Add the coconut flour, baking powder, salt, cheese and Italian seasoning. Combine until the ingredients are well combined. Add more flour if the mixture is too thick.

3. Pour an appropriate amount of the batter into the waffle maker and spread out the batter to cover all the holes on the waffle maker.

4. Cover the waffle maker and cook for about 7 minutes or according to your waffle maker's settings. Make sure the chaffle is browned.

5. After the cooking cycle, use a plastic or silicone utensil to remove the chaffle form the waffle maker.

6. Repeat step 3 to 5 until you have cooked all the batter into chaffles.

7. Cut the chaffles into sticks. Each mini chaffle should make about 4 sticks.

8. Preheat the oven to 350°F. Line a baking sheet with parchment paper and grease it with the melted butter.

9. Break the remaining two eggs into another mixing bowl and beat.

10. In another mixing bowl, combine the oregano, pepper, garlic and onion.

11. Dip one chaffle stick into the egg. Bring it out and hold it for a few seconds to allow excess liquid to drip off.

12. Dip the wet chaffle stick into the seasoning mixture and make sure it is coated with seasoning. Drop it on the baking sheet.

13. Repeat step 11 and 12 until all the

chaffle sticks are coated.

14. Arrange the chaffle sticks into the baking sheet in a single layer.

15. Place the baking sheet in the oven and bake for 10 minutes.

16. Remove the baking sheet from the oven, brush the oil over the sticks and flip them.

17. Return it to the oven and bake for an additional 6 minutes or until the stick are golden brown.

18. Remove the sticks from the oven and let them cool for a few minutes.

19. Serve and enjoy.

402. Cinnamon Roll Chaffle

Preparation time: 7 mins
Cooking time: 9 mins
Servings: 3

Ingredients:

- 1 egg (beaten)
- ½ cup shredded mozzarella cheese
- 1 tsp cinnamon
- 1 tsp sugar free maple syrup
- ¼ tsp baking powder
- 1 tbsp almond flour
- ½ tsp vanilla extract
- Topping:
- 2 tsp granulated swerve
- 1 tbsp heavy cream
- 4 tbsp cream cheese

Directions:

1. Plug the waffle maker to preheat it and spray it with a non-stick spray.

2. In a mixing bowl, whisk together the egg, maple syrup and vanilla extract.

3. In another mixing bowl, combine the cinnamon, almond flour, baking powder and mozzarella cheese.

4. Pour in the egg mixture into the flour mixture and mix until the ingredients are well combined.

5. Pour in an appropriate amount of the batter into the waffle maker and spread out the batter to the edges to cover all the holes on the waffle maker.

6. Close the waffle maker and bake for about 3 minute or according to your waffle maker's settings.

7. After the cooking cycle, use a silicone or plastic utensil to remove the chaffle from the waffle maker.

8. Repeat step 5 to 7 until you have cooked all the batter into chaffles.

9. For the topping, combine the cream cheese, swerve and heavy cream in a microwave safe dish.

10. Place the dish in a microwave and microwave on high until the mixture is melted and smooth. Stir every 15 seconds.

11. Top the chaffles with the cream mixture and enjoy.

403. Cereal and walnut Chaffle

Preparation time: 5 mins
Cooking time: 6 mins
Servings: 2

Ingredients:

- 1 milliliter of cereal flavoring
- ¼ tsp baking powder
- 1 tsp granulated swerve
- 1/8 tsp xanthan gum
- 1 tbsp butter (melted)
- ½ tsp coconut flour

- 2 tbsp toasted walnut (chopped)
- 1 tbsp cream cheese
- 2 tbsp almond flour
- 1 large egg (beaten)
- ¼ tsp cinnamon
- 1/8 tsp nutmeg

Directions:

1. Plug the waffle maker to preheat it and spray it with a non-stick spray.
2. In a mixing bowl, whisk together the egg, cereal flavoring, cream cheese and butter.
3. In another mixing bowl, combine the coconut flour, almond flour, cinnamon, nutmeg, swerve, xanthan gum and baking powder.
4. Pour the egg mixture into the flour mixture and mix until you form a smooth batter.
5. Fold in the chopped walnuts.
6. Pour in an appropriate amount of the batter into the waffle maker and spread out the batter to the edges to cover all the holes on the waffle maker.
7. Close the waffle maker and cook for about 3 minutes or according to your waffle maker's settings.
8. After the cooking cycle, use a plastic or silicone utensil to remove the chaffle from the waffle maker.
9. Repeat step 6 to 8 until you have cooked all the batter into chaffles.
10. Serve and top with sour cream or heavy cream.

404. Beef Zucchini Chaffle

Preparation time: 10 minutes
Cooking time: 5 minutes
Servings: 2

Ingredients:

- Zucchini: 1 (small)
- Beef: ½ cup boneless
- Egg: 1
- Shredded mozzarella: half cup
- Pepper: as per your taste
- Salt: as per your taste
- Basil: 1 tsp

Directions:

1. Boil beef in water to make it tender
2. Shred it into small pieces and set aside
3. Preheat your waffle iron
4. Grate zucchini finely
5. Add all the ingredients to zucchini in a bowl and mix well
6. Now add the shredded beef
7. Grease your waffle iron lightly
8. Pour the mixture into a full-size waffle maker and spread evenly
9. Cook till it turns crispy
10. Make as many chaffles as your mixture and waffle maker allow
11. Serve crispy and with your favorite keto sauce

405. Spinach Beef Chaffle

Preparation time: 10 minutes
Cooking time: 5 minutes
Servings: 2

Ingredients:

- Spinach: ½ cup
- Beef: ½ cup boneless
- Egg: 1
- Shredded mozzarella: half cup

- Pepper: as per your taste
- Garlic powder: 1 tbsp
- Salt: as per your taste
- Basil: 1 tsp

Directions:

1. Boil beef in water to make it tender
2. Shred it into small pieces and set aside
3. Boil spinach in a saucepan for 10 minutes and strain
4. Preheat your waffle iron
5. Add all the ingredients to boiled spinach in a bowl and mix well
6. Now add the shredded beef
7. Grease your waffle iron lightly
8. Pour the mixture into a full-size waffle maker and spread evenly
9. Cook till it turns crispy
10. Make as many chaffles as your mixture and waffle maker allow
11. Serve crispy and with your favorite keto sauce

406. Crispy Beef Burger Chaffle

Preparation time: 20 minutes
Cooking time: 10 minutes
Servings: 2

Ingredients:

- For the chaffle:
- Egg: 2
- Mozzarella cheese: 1 cup (shredded)
- Butter: 1 tbsp
- Almond flour: 2 tbsp
- Baking powder: ¼ tsp
- Onion powder: a pinch
- Garlic powder: a pinch

- Salt: a pinch
- For the beef:
- Ground beef: 1 lb
- Chives: 2 tbsp
- Cheddar cheese: 1 cup
- Salt: ¼ tsp or as per your taste
- Black pepper: ¼ tsp or as per your taste

Directions:

1. Mix all the beef ingredient in a bowl
2. Make patties either grill them or fry them
3. Preheat a mini waffle maker if needed and grease it
4. In a mixing bowl, add all the chaffle ingredients and mix well
5. Pour the mixture to the lower plate of the waffle maker and spread it evenly to cover the plate properly and close the lid
6. Cook for at least 4 minutes to get the desired crunch
7. Remove the chaffle from the heat and keep aside for around one minute
8. Make as many chaffles as your mixture and waffle maker allow
9. Serve with the beef patties in between two chaffles

407. Crispy Beef Artichoke Chaffle

Preparation time: 10 minutes
Cooking time: 5 minutes
Servings: 2

Ingredients:

- Beef: ½ cup cooked grounded
- Artichokes: 1 cup chopped
- Egg: 1

- Mozzarella cheese: 1/2 cup (shredded)
- Cream cheese: 1 ounce
- Salt: as per your taste
- Garlic powder: ¼ tsp
- Onion powder: ¼ tsp

Directions:

1. Preheat a mini waffle maker if needed and grease it
2. In a mixing bowl, add all the ingredients
3. Mix them all well
4. Pour the mixture to the lower plate of the waffle maker and spread it evenly to cover the plate properly
5. Close the lid
6. Cook for at least 4 minutes to get the desired crunch
7. Remove the chaffle from the heat and keep aside for around one minute
8. Make as many chaffles as your mixture and waffle maker allow
9. Serve hot with your favorite keto sauce

408. Beef Cheddar Chaffle

Preparation time: 15 minutes
Cooking time: 8 minutes
Servings: 2
Ingredients:

- Beef: 1 cup (grounder)
- Egg: 2
- Chedder cheese: 1 cup
- Mozarrella cheese: 4 tbsp
- Tomato sauce: 6 tbsp
- Basil: ½ tsp
- Garlic: ½ tbsp

- Butter: 1 tsp

Directions:

1. In a pan, add butter and include beef
2. Stir for two minutes and then add garlic and basil
3. Cook till tender
4. Set aside the cooked beef
5. Preheat the mini waffle maker if needed
6. Mix cooked beef, eggs, and 1 cup mozzarella cheese properly
7. Spread it to the mini waffle maker thoroughly
8. Cook for 4 minutes or till it turns crispy and then remove it from the waffle maker
9. Make as many mini chaffles as you can
10. Now in a baking tray, line these mini chaffles and top with the tomato sauce and grated mozzarella cheese
11. Put the tray in the oven at 400 degrees until the cheese melts
12. Serve hot with your favorite keto sauce

409. Beef Broccoli Chaffle

Preparation time: 10 minutes
Cooking time: 5 minutes
Servings: 2

Ingredients:

- Broccoli: ½ cup
- Beef: ½ cup boneless
- Butter: 2 tbsp
- Egg: 1
- Shredded mozzarella: half cup
- Pepper: as per your taste

- Garlic powder: 1 tbsp
- Salt: as per your taste
- Basil: 1 tsp

Directions:

1. In a pan, add butter and include beef
2. Stir for two minutes and then add garlic and basil
3. Cook till tender
4. Boil broccoli for 10 minutes in a separate pan and blend
5. Set aside the cooked beef
6. Preheat the mini waffle maker if needed
7. Mix cooked beef, broccoli blend, eggs, and 1 cup mozzarella cheese properly
8. Spread it to the mini waffle maker thoroughly
9. Cook for 4 minutes or till it turns crispy and then remove it from the waffle maker
10. Make as many mini chaffles as you can
11. Now in a baking tray, line these mini chaffles and top with the tomato sauce and grated mozzarella cheese
12. Put the tray in the oven at 400 degrees until the cheese melts
13. Serve hot with your favorite keto sauce

410. Garlic Lobster Chaffle Roll

Preparation time: 5 minutes
Cooking time: 5 minutes
Servings: 2

Ingredients:

- For chaffle:
- Egg: 2

- Mozzarella cheese: 1 cup (shredded)
- Bay seasoning: ½ tsp
- Garlic powder: ¼ tsp
- For lobster mix:
- Langostino tails: 1 cup
- Kewpie mayo: 2 tbsp
- Garlic powder: ½ tsp
- Lemon juice: 2 tsp
- Parsley: 1 tsp (chopped) for garnishing

Directions:

1. Defrost langostino tails
2. In a small mixing bowl, mix langostino tails with lemon juice, garlic powder, and kewpie mayo; mix properly and keep aside
3. In another mixing bowl, beat eggs and add mozzarella cheese to them with garlic powder and bay seasoning
4. Mix them all well and pour to the greasy mini waffle maker
5. Cook for at least 4 minutes to get the desired crunch
6. Remove the chaffle from the heat, add the lobster mixture in between and fold
7. Make as many chaffles as your mixture and waffle maker allow
8. Serve hot and enjoy!

411. Fried Fish Chaffles

Preparation time: 15 minutes
Cooking time: 10 minutes
Servings: 2

Ingredients:

- For chaffle:
- Egg: 2

- Mozzarella cheese: 1 cup (shredded)
- Bay seasoning: ½ tsp
- Garlic powder: ¼ tsp
- For fried fish:
- Fish boneless: 1 cup
- Garlic powder: 1 tbsp
- Onion powder: 1 tbsp
- Salt: ¼ tsp or as per your taste
- Black pepper: ¼ tsp or as per your taste
- Turmeric: ¼ tsp
- Red chili flakes: ½ tbsp
- Butter: 2 tbsp

Directions:

1. Marinate the fish with all the ingredients of the fried fish except for butter
2. Melt butter in a medium-size frying pan and add the marinated fish
3. Fry from both sides for at least 5 minutes and set aside
4. Preheat a mini waffle maker if needed and grease it
5. In a mixing bowl, beat eggs and add all the chaffle ingredients
6. Mix them all well
7. Pour the mixture to the lower plate of the waffle maker and spread it evenly to cover the plate properly
8. Close the lid
9. Cook for at least 4 minutes to get the desired crunch
10. Remove the chaffle from the heat and keep aside for around one minute
11. Make as many chaffles as your mixture and waffle maker allow
12. Serve hot with the prepared fish

412. Crispy Crab Chaffle

Preparation time: 25 minutes
Cooking time: 10 minutes
Servings: 2

Ingredients:

- For chaffle:
- Egg: 1
- Mozzarella cheese: ½ cup (shredded)
- Salt: ¼ tsp or as per your taste
- Black pepper: ¼ tsp or as per your taste
- Ginger powder: 1 tbsp
- For crab
- Crab meat: 1 cup
- Butter: 2 tbsp
- Salt: ¼ tsp or as per your taste
- Black pepper: ¼ tsp or as per your taste
- Red chili flakes: ½ tsp

Directions:

1. In a frying pan, melt butter and fry crab meat for two minutes
2. Add the spices at the end and set aside
3. Mix all the chaffle ingredients well together
4. Pour a thin layer on a preheated waffle iron
5. Add prepared crab and pour again more mixture over the top
6. Cook the chaffle for around 5 minutes
7. Make as many chaffles as your mixture and waffle maker allow
8. Serve hot with your favorite sauce

413. Simple Cabbage Chaffles

Preparation time: 10 minutes
Cooking time: 5 minutes
Servings: 2

Ingredients:

- Egg: 2
- Mozzarella cheese: 1 cup (shredded)
- Butter: 2 tbsp
- Almond flour: 2 tbsp
- Turmeric: ¼ tsp
- Baking powder: ¼ tsp
- Onion powder: a pinch
- Garlic powder: a pinch
- Salt: as per your taste
- cabbage: 1 cup shredded

Directions:

1. Take a frying pan and melt 1 tbsp of butter
2. Add the shredded cabbage and sauté for 4 minutes and set aside
3. In a mixing bowl, add all the ingredients and mix well
4. Pour a thin layer on a preheated waffle iron
5. Add cabbage on top of the mixture
6. Again add more mixture over the top
7. Cook the chaffle for around 5 minutes
8. Serve hot with your favorite keto sauce

414. Cabbage and Artichoke Chaffle

Preparation time: 10 minutes
Cooking time: 5 minutes
Servings: 2

Ingredients:

- Artichokes: 1/2 cup chopped
- Cabbage: ½ cup

- Black pepper: ½ tbsp
- Egg: 1
- Mozzarella cheese: 1/2 cup (shredded)
- Cream cheese: 1 ounce
- Salt: as per your taste
- Garlic powder: ¼ tsp
- Turmeric: ¼ tsp
- baking powder: ¼ tsp

Directions:

1. Take a frying pan and melt 1 tbsp of butter
2. Add the shredded cabbage and sauté for 4 minutes and set aside
3. In a mixing bowl, add all the ingredients and mix well
4. Pour a thin layer on a preheated waffle iron
5. Add cabbage on top of the mixture
6. Again add more mixture over the top
7. Cook the chaffle for around 5 minutes
8. Serve hot with your favorite keto sauce

415. Zucchini BBQ Chaffle

Preparation time: 10 minutes
Cooking time: 5 minutes
Servings: 2

Ingredients:

- Zucchini: 1/2 cup
- Bbq sauce: 1 tbsp (sugar-free)
- Almond flour: 2 tbsp
- Egg: 1
- Cheddar cheese: ½ cup

Directions:

1. Finely grate zucchini

2. Preheat your waffle iron

3. In mixing bowl, add all the chaffle ingredients including zucchini and mix well

4. Grease your waffle iron lightly

5. Pour the mixture to the bottom plate evenly; also spread it out to get better results and close the upper plate and heat

6. Cook for 6 minutes or until the chaffle is done

7. Make as many chaffles as your mixture and waffle maker allow

416. Eggplant BBQ Chaffle

Preparation time: 10 minutes
Cooking time: 5 minutes
Servings: 2

Ingredients:

- Egg plant: 1/2 cup
- Bbq sauce: 1 tbsp (sugar-free)
- Almond flour: 2 tbsp
- Egg: 1
- cheddar cheese: ½ cup

Directions:

1. Boil egg plant in water, and strain

2. Preheat your waffle iron

3. In mixing bowl, add all the chaffle ingredients including zucchini and mix well

4. Grease your waffle iron lightly

5. Pour the mixture to the bottom plate evenly; also spread it out to get better results and close the upper plate and heat

6. Cook for 6 minutes or until the chaffle is done

7. Make as many chaffles as your mixture and waffle maker allow

417. Zucchini Olives Chaffles

Preparation time: 10 minutes
Cooking time: 5 minutes
Servings: 2

Ingredients:

- Egg: 2
- Mozzarella cheese: 1 cup (shredded)
- Butter: 1 tbsp
- Almond flour: 2 tbsp
- Turmeric: ¼ tsp
- Baking powder: ¼ tsp
- Onion powder: a pinch
- Garlic powder: a pinch
- Salt: a pinch
- black pepper: ¼ tsp or as per your taste
- spinach: ½ cup
- olives: 5-10

Directions:

1. Boil the spinach in water for around 10 minutes and drain the remaining water

2. In a mixing bowl, add all the above-mentioned ingredients except for olives

3. Mix well and add the boils spinach

4. Pour the mixture to the lower plate of the waffle maker and spread it evenly to cover the plate properly

5. Sprinkle the sliced olives as per choice over the mixture and close the lid

6. Cook for at least 4 minutes to get the desired crunch

7. Remove the chaffle from the heat

8. Make as many chaffles as your mixture and waffle maker allow

9. Serve hot and enjoy!

418. Cauliflower Mozzarella Chaffle

Preparation time: 15 minutes
Cooking time: 8 minutes
Servings: 2

Ingredients:

- Cauliflower: 1 cup
- Egg: 2
- Mozzarella cheese: 1 cup and 4 tbsp
- Tomato sauce: 6 tbsp
- Basil: ½ tsp
- Garlic: ½ tbsp
- Butter: 1 tsp

Directions:

1. In a pan, add butter and include small pieces of cauliflower to it
2. Stir for two minutes and then add garlic and basil
3. Set aside the cooked cauliflower
4. Preheat the mini waffle maker if needed
5. Mix cooked cauliflower, eggs, and 1 cup mozzarella cheese properly
6. Spread it to the mini waffle maker thoroughly
7. Cook for 4 minutes or till it turns crispy and then remove it from the waffle maker
8. Make as many mini chaffles as you can
9. Now in a baking tray, line these mini chaffles and top with the tomato sauce and grated mozzarella cheese
10. Put the tray in the oven at 400 degrees until the cheese melts
11. Serve hot

419. Plain Artichok Chaffle

Preparation time: 10 minutes
Cooking time: 5 minutes
Servings: 2

Ingredients:

- Artichokes: 1 cup chopped
- Egg: 1
- Mozzarella cheese: 1/2 cup (shredded)
- Cream cheese: 1 ounce
- Salt: as per your taste
- Garlic powder: ¼ tsp

Directions:

1. Preheat a mini waffle maker if needed and grease it
2. In a mixing bowl, add all the ingredients
3. Mix them all well
4. Pour the mixture to the lower plate of the waffle maker and spread it evenly to cover the plate properly
5. Close the lid
6. Cook for at least 4 minutes to get the desired crunch
7. Remove the chaffle from the heat and keep aside for around one minute
8. Make as many chaffles as your mixture and waffle maker allow
9. Serve hot with your favorite keto sauce

CAKE AND SNACKS

420 Pecan Pie Cake Chaffle:

Preparation Time: 15 minutes
Cooking Time: 25 minutes
Servings: 2

Ingredients:

- For Pecan Pie Chaffle:
- Egg: 1
- Cream cheese: 2 tbsp
- Maple extract: ½ tbsp
- Almond flour: 4 tbsp
- Sukrin Gold: 1 tbsp
- Baking powder: ½ tbsp
- Pecan: 2 tbsp chopped
- Heavy whipping cream: 1 tbsp
- For Pecan Pie Filling:
- Butter: 2 tbsp
- Sukrin Gold: 1 tbsp
- Pecan: 2 tbsp chopped
- Heavy whipping cream: 2 tbsp
- Maple syrup: 2 tbsp
- Egg yolk: 2 large
- Salt: a pinch

Directions:

1. In a small saucepan, add sweetener, butter, syrups, and heavy whipping cream and use a low flame to heat
2. Mix all the ingredients well together
3. Remove from heat and add egg yolks and mix
4. Now put it on heat again and stir
5. Add pecan and salt to the mixture and let it simmer
6. It will thicken then remove from heat and let it rest
7. For the chaffles, add all the ingredients except pecans and blend
8. Now add pecan with a spoon
9. Preheat a mini waffle maker if needed and grease it
10. Pour the mixture to the lower plate of the waffle maker and spread it evenly to cover the plate properly and close the lid
11. Cook for at least 4 minutes to get the desired crunch
12. Remove the chaffle from the heat and keep aside for around one minute
13. Make as many chaffles as your mixture and waffle maker allow
14. Add 1/3 the previously prepared pecan pie filling to the chaffle and arrange like a cake

422. German Chocolate Chaffle Cake:

Preparation Time: 5 minutes
Cooking Time: 10 minutes
Servings: 2

Ingredients:

- For Chocolate Chaffle:
- Egg: 1
- Cream cheese: 2 tbsp
- Powdered sweetener: 1 tbsp
- Vanilla extract: ½ tbsp
- Instant coffee powder: ¼ tsp
- Almond flour: 1 tbsp

- Cocoa powder: 1 tbsp (unsweetened)
- For Filling:
- Egg Yolk: 1
- Heavy cream: ¼ cup
- Butter: 1 tbsp
- Powdered sweetener: 2 tbsp
- Caramel: ½ tsp
- Coconut flakes: ¼ cup
- Coconut flour: 1 tsp
- Pecans: ¼ cups chopped

Directions:

1. Preheat a mini waffle maker if needed and grease it
2. In a mixing bowl, beat eggs and add the remaining chaffle ingredients
3. Mix them all well
4. Pour the mixture to the lower plate of the waffle maker and spread it evenly to cover the plate properly and close the lid
5. Cook for at least 4 minutes to get the desired crunch
6. Remove the chaffle from the heat and let them cool completely
7. Make as many chaffles as your mixture and waffle maker allow
8. In a small pan, mix heavy cream, egg yolk, sweetener, and butter at low heat for around 5 minutes
9. Remove from heat and add the remaining ingredients to make the filling
10. Stack chaffles on one another and add filling in between to enjoy the cake

422. Almond Chocolate Chaffle Cake:

Preparation Time: 5 minutes

Cooking Time: 10 minutes
Servings: 2

Ingredients:

- For Chocolate Chaffle:
- Egg: 1
- Cream cheese: 2 tbsp
- Powdered sweetener: 1 tbsp
- Vanilla extract: ½ tbsp
- Instant coffee powder: ¼ tsp
- Almond flour: 1 tbsp
- Cocoa powder: 1 tbsp (unsweetened)
- For Coconut Filling:
- Melted Coconut Oil: 1 ½ tbsp
- Heavy cream: 1 tbsp
- Cream cheese: 4 tbsp
- Powdered sweetener: 1 tbsp
- Vanilla extract: ½ tbsp
- Coconut: ¼ cup finely shredded
- Whole almonds: 14

Directions:

1. Preheat a mini waffle maker if needed and grease it
2. In a mixing bowl, add all the chaffle ingredients
3. Mix them all well
4. Pour the mixture to the lower plate of the waffle maker and spread it evenly to cover the plate properly
5. Close the lid
6. Cook for at least 4 minutes to get the desired crunch
7. Remove the chaffle from the heat and keep aside for around one minute
8. Make as many chaffles as your mixture and waffle maker allow

9. Except for almond, add all the filling ingredients in a bowl and mix well

10. Spread the filling on the chaffle and spread almonds on top with another chaffle at almonds – stack the chaffles and fillings like a cake and enjoy

423. Carrot Cake Chaffle

Preparation Time: 10 minutes
Cooking Time: 15 minutes
Servings: 2

Ingredients:

- For Carrot Chaffle Cake:
- Carrot: ½ cup (shredded)
- Egg: 1
- Heavy whipping cream: 2 tbsp
- Butter: 2 tbsp (melted)
- Powdered sweetener: 2 tbsp
- Walnuts: 1 tbsp (chopped)
- Almond flour: ¾ cup
- Cinnamon powder: 2 tsp
- Baking powder: 1 tsp
- Pumpkin sauce: 1 tsp
- For Cream Cheese Frosting:
- Cream cheese: ½ cup
- Heavy whipping cream: 2 tbsp
- Vanilla extract: 1 tsp
- Powdered sweetener: ¼ cup

Directions:

- Mix all the ingredients together one by one until they form a uniform consistency
- Preheat a mini waffle maker if needed and grease it
- Pour the mixture to the lower plate of the waffle maker

- Close the lid
- Cook for at least 4 minutes to get the desired crunch
- Prepare frosting by combining all the ingredients of the cream cheese frosting using a hand mixer
- Remove the chaffle from the heat and keep aside for around a few minutes
- Make as many chaffles as your mixture and waffle maker allow
- Stack the chaffles with frosting in between in such a way that it gives the look of a cake

424. Peanut Butter Keto Chaffle Cake

Preparation Time: 5 minutes
Cooking Time: 10 minutes
Servings: 2

Ingredients:

- For Chaffles:
- Egg: 1
- Peanut Butter:: 2 tbsp (sugar-free)
- Monkfruit: 2 tbsp
- Baking powder: ¼ tsp
- Peanut butter extract: ¼ tsp
- Heavy whipping cream: 1 tsp
- For Peanut Butter Frosting:
- Monkfruit: 2 tsp
- Cream cheese: 2 tbsp
- Butter: 1 tbsp
- Peanut butter: 1 tbsp (sugar-free)
- Vanilla: ¼ tsp

Directions:

1. Preheat a mini waffle maker if needed and grease it

2. In a mixing bowl, beat eggs and add all the chaffle ingredients

3. Mix them all well and pour the mixture to the lower plate of the waffle maker

4. Close the lid

5. Cook for at least 4 minutes to get the desired crunch

6. Remove the chaffle from the heat and keep aside for around a few minutes

7. Make as many chaffles as your mixture and waffle maker allow

8. In a separate bowl, add all the frosting ingredients and whisk well to give it a uniform consistency

9. Assemble chaffles in a way that in between two chaffles you put the frosting and make the cake

425. Strawberry Shortcake Chaffle

Preparation Time: 5 minutes
Cooking Time: 10 minutes
Servings: 2

Ingredients:

- Egg: 1
- Heavy Whipping Cream: 1 tbsp
- Any non-sugar sweetener: 2 tbsp
- Coconut Flour: 1 tsp
- Cake batter extract: ½ tsp
- Baking powder: ¼ tsp
- Strawberry: 4 or as per your taste

Directions:

1. Preheat a mini waffle maker if needed and grease it

2. In a mixing bowl, beat eggs and add non-sugar sweetener, coconut flour, baking powder, and cake batter extract

3. Mix them all well and pour the mixture to the lower plate of the waffle maker

4. Close the lid

5. Cook for at least 4 minutes to get the desired crunch

6. Remove the chaffle from the heat and keep aside for around two minutes

7. Make as many chaffles as your mixture and waffle maker allow

8. Serve with whipped cream and strawberries on top

426. Italian Cream Chaffle Cake

Preparation Time: 8 minutes
Cooking Time: 12 minutes
Servings: 3

Ingredients:

- For Chaffle:
- Egg: 4
- Mozzarella Cheese: ½ cup
- Almond flour: 1 tbsp
- Coconut flour: 4 tbsp
- Monkfruit sweetener: 1 tbsp
- Vanilla extract: 1 tsp
- Baking powder: 1 ½ tsp
- Cinnamon powder: ½ tsp
- Butter: 1 tbsp (melted)
- Coconut: 1 tsp (shredded)
- Walnuts: 1 tsp (chopped)
- For Italian Cream Frosting:
- Cream cheese: 4 tbsp
- Butter: 2 tbsp
- Vanilla: ½ tsp
- Monkfruit sweetener: 2 tbs

Directions:

1. Blend eggs, cream cheese, sweetener, vanilla, coconut flour, melted butter, almond flour, and baking powder
2. Make the mixture creamy
3. Preheat a mini waffle maker if needed and grease it
4. Pour the mixture to the lower plate of the waffle maker
5. Close the lid
6. Cook for at least 4 minutes to get the desired crunch
7. Remove the chaffle from the heat and keep aside to cool it
8. Make as many chaffles as your mixture and waffle maker allow
9. Garnish with shredded coconut and chopped walnuts

427. Banana Cake Pudding Chaffle

Preparation Time: 10 minutes
Cooking Time: 1 hour
Servings: 2

Ingredients:

- For Banana Chaffle:
- Cream cheese: 2 tbsp
- Banana extract: 1 tsp
- Mozzarella cheese: ¼ cup
- Egg: 1
- Sweetener: 2 tbsp
- Almond flour: 4 tbsp
- Baking powder: 1 tsp
- For Banana Pudding:
- Egg yolk: 1 large
- Powdered sweetener: 3 tbsp
- Xanthan gum: ½ tsp
- Heavy whipping cream: 1/2 cup
- Banana extract: ½ tsp
- Salt: a pinch

Directions:

1. In a pan, add powdered sweetener, heavy cream, and egg yolk and whisk continuously so the mixture thickens
2. Simmer for a minute only
3. Add xanthan gum to the mixture and whisk again
4. Remove the pan from heat and add banana extract and salt and mix them all well
5. Shift the mixture to a glass dish and refrigerate the pudding
6. Preheat a mini waffle maker if needed and grease it
7. In a mixing bowl, add all the chaffle ingredients
8. Mix them all well and pour the mixture to the lower plate of the waffle maker
9. Close the lid
10. Cook for at least 5 minutes to get the desired crunch
11. Remove the chaffle from the heat and keep aside for around a few minutes
12. Stack chaffles and pudding one by one to form a cake

428. Cream Coconut Chaffle Cake

Preparation Time: 20 minutes
Cooking Time: 1 hour 20 minutes (depends on your refrigerator)
Servings: 2

Ingredients:

- For Chaffles:
- Egg: 2

- Powdered sweetener: 2 tbsp
- Cream cheese: 2 tbsp
- Vanilla extract: 1/2 tsp
- Butter: 1 tbsp (melted)
- Coconut: 2 tbsp (shredded)
- Coconut extract: ½ tsp
- For Filling:
- Coconut: ¼ cup (shredded)
- Butter: 2 tsp
- Monkfruit sweetener: 2 tbsp
- Xanthan gum: ¼ tsp
- Salt: a pinch
- Egg yolks: 2
- Almond: 1/3 cup unsweetened
- Coconut milk: 1/3 cup
- For Garnishing:
- Whipped Cream: as per your taste
- Coconut: 1 tbsp (shredded)

Directions:

1. Preheat a mini waffle maker if needed and grease it
2. In a mixing bowl, add all the chaffle ingredients
3. Mix them all well and pour the mixture to the lower plate of the waffle maker
4. Close the lid
5. Cook for at least 4 minutes to get the desired crunch
6. Remove the chaffle from the heat and keep aside for around a few minutes
7. Make as many chaffles as your mixture and waffle maker allow
8. For the filling, in a small pan, cook almond milk and coconut together on medium heat in such way that it only steams but doesn't boil
9. In another bowl, lightly whish egg yolks and add milk to it continuously
10. Heat the mixture so it thickens, again it must not boil
11. Add sweetener and whisk while adding Xanthan Gum bit by bit
12. Remove from heat and mix all the other ingredients
13. Mix well and refrigerate; the mixture will further thicken when cool
14. Assemble the prepared chaffles and cream on top of one another to make the cake-like shape
15. Garnish with coconuts and whipped cream at the end

429. Lemon Chaffle Cake

Preparation Time: 40 minutes (depends on chaffle's cooling)
Cooking Time: 20 minutes
Servings: 2

Ingredients:

- For Chaffles:
- Egg: 2
- Powdered sweetener: 1 tbsp
- Cream cheese: 4 tbsp
- Butter: 2 tbsp (melted)
- Coconut flour: 2 tsp
- Baking powder: 1 tsp
- Lemon extract: ½ tsp
- Cake batter extract: 20 drops
- For Frosting:
- Heavy whipping cream: ½ cup
- Monkfruit sweetener: 1 tbsp
- Lemon extract: ¼ tsp

Directions:

1. Preheat a mini waffle maker if needed and grease it

2. In a blender, add all the chaffle ingredients and blend

3. Pour the mixture to the lower plate of the waffle maker and spread it evenly to cover the plate properly

4. Close the lid

5. Cook for at least 4 minutes to get the desired crunch

6. Remove the chaffle from the heat and keep aside

7. Make as many chaffles as your mixture and waffle maker allow

8. Prepare the frosting by whisking all the frosting ingredients till it thickens and attains uniform consistency

9. When all the chaffles cool down, arrange in the form of cake by adding frosting in between

430. Keto Birthday Chaffle Cake

Preparation Time: 40 minutes
Cooking Time: 20 minutes
Servings: 2

Ingredients:

- For Chaffle:
- Egg: 2
- Powdered sweetener: 2 tbsp
- Cream cheese: 2 tbsp
- Butter: 2 tbsp (melted)
- Coconut flour: 2 tsp
- Almond flour: ¼ cup
- Baking powder: ½ tsp
- Vanilla extract: ½ tsp
- Xanthan powder ¼ tsp

- For Frosting:
- Heavy whipping cream: 1/2 cup
- Swerve: 2 tbsp
- Vanilla extract: ½ tsp

Directions:

1. Preheat a mini waffle maker if needed

2. In a medium-size blender, add all the cake ingredients and blend till it forms a creamy texture

3. Let the batter sit for a minute or two; appearance is watery but it produces crunchy chaffles

4. Pour the batter to the lower plate of the waffle maker and spread it evenly to cover the plate properly

5. Close the lid

6. Cook for at least 4 minutes to get the desired crunch

7. Remove the chaffle from the heat and keep aside to cool totally

8. For the frosting, add all the ingredients in a bowl and use a hand mixer until the cream thickens

9. Make as many chaffles as your mixture and waffle maker allow

10. Frost the chaffles in a way you like

11. Serve cool and enjoy!

431. Tiramasu Chaffle Cake:

Preparation Time: 20 minutes
Cooking Time: 40 minutes
Servings: 4

Ingredients:

- Egg: 2
- Monkfruit sweetener: 2 tbsp
- Cream cheese: 2 tbsp
- Butter: 2 tbsp (melted)

- Coconut flour: 2 tbsp
- Baking powder: 1 tsp
- Vanilla extract: ½ tsp
- Instant coffee dry mix: 2 ½ tsp

- Hazelnut extract: ½ tsp
- Almond flour: ¼ cup
- Organic cacao powder: 1 ½ tbsp
- Himalayan pink fine salt: 1/8 tsp
- Mascarpone Cheese: ½ cup
- Powdered sweetener: ¼ cup

Directions:

1. In a microwave, melt butter for a minute and then add instant coffee, stir it continuously

2. In a bowl, beat eggs, cream cheese and the butter-coffee mixture

3. In a separate bowl, add sweetener, vanilla extract, and mascarpone cheese

4. In the egg mixture, add all the dry ingredients into it and mix well

5. Preheat a mini waffle maker if needed and grease it

6. Pour the egg mixture to the lower plate of the waffle maker and spread it evenly to cover the plate properly and close the lid

7. Cook for at least 4 minutes to get the desired crunch

8. Remove the chaffle from the heat and keep aside to cool down

9. Make as many chaffles as your mixture and waffle maker allow

10. If you want to have two layers cake then split the cream

11. You can also separate cacao powder ½ tbsp and instant coffee ½ tsp and blend

12. Layer the cake in a way that spread cream and coffee mixture on one chaffle and add another chaffle on top

13. Serve cool and enjoy!

432. Birthday Cake Chaffle

Preparation time: 10 minutes
Cooking time: 12 minutes
Servings: 2

Ingredients:

- 1 egg (beaten)
- 2 tbsp almond flour
- 1 tbsp swerve sweetener
- ½ tsp cake batter extract
- ¼ tsp baking powder
- 1 tbsp heavy whipping cream
- 2 tbsp cream cheese
- ½ tsp vanilla extract
- ½ tsp cinnamon
- Frosting:
- 1 tbsp swerve
- ¼ cup heavy whipping cream
- ½ tsp vanilla extract

Directions:

1. Plug the waffle maker to preheat it and spray it with a non-stick spray.

2. In a mixing bowl, combine the cinnamon, almond flour, baking

powder and swerve.

3. In another mixing bowl, whisk together the egg, vanilla, heavy cream, and cake batter extract.

4. Pour the flour mixture into the egg mixture and mix until the ingredients are well combined and you have formed a smooth batter.

5. Pour an appropriate amount of the batter into the waffle maker and spread out the waffle maker to cover all the holes on the waffle maker.

6. Close the waffle maker and bake for about 3 minutes or according to your waffle maker's settings.

7. After the cooking cycle, use a silicone or plastic utensil to remove the chaffle from the waffle maker.

8. Repeat step 5 to 7 until you have cooked all the batter into chaffles.

9. For the cream, whisk together the swerve, heavy cream and vanilla extract until smooth and fluffy.

10. To assemble the cake, place one chaffle on a flat surface and spread 1/3 of the cream over it. Layer another chaffle on the first one and spread 1/3 of the cream over it too. Repeat this for the last chaffle and the remaining cream.

Cut cake and serve.

433. Chocolate Chaffle Cake

Preparation Time: 2 minutes
Cooking Time: 8 minutes
Servings: 2

Ingredients

- 2 tablespoons cocoa powder

- 2 tablespoons swerve granulated sugar

- 1 egg

- 1 tablespoon overwhelming whipping cream

- 1 tablespoon almond flour

- 1/4 tsp preparing powder

- 1/2 tsp vanilla concentrate

Directions:

1. Add all the recipes together to get the exact formula

434. Keto Blueberry Waffles

Preparation Time: 3 minutes
Cooking Time: 15 minutes
Servings: 5

Ingredients

- 1 cup of mozzarella cheddar

- 2 tablespoons almond flour

- 1 tsp heating powder

- 2 eggs

- 1 tsp cinnamon

- 2 tsp of Swerve

- 3 tablespoon blueberries

Directions

1. Heat up your Dash smaller than expected waffle producer.

2. In a blending, bowl includes the mozzarella cheddar, almond flour, heating powder, eggs, cinnamon, swerve and blueberries. Blend well so every one of the fixings is combined.

3. Spray your smaller than expected waffle producer with nonstick cooking shower.

4. Add shortly less than 1/4 a cup of blueberry keto waffle player.

5. Close the top and cook the chaffle for 3-5 minutes. Check it at the brief imprint to check whether it is firm

and dark-colored. In the event that it isn't or it adheres to the highest point of the waffle machine close the cover and cook for 1-2 minutes longer.

6. Serve with a sprinkle of swerve confectioners sugar or keto syrup.

435. Keto Pizza Chaffle

Preparation time: 15 minutes
Cooking time: 6 minutes

Ingredients

- 1 tsp coconut flour
- 1 egg white
- 1/2 cup mozzarella cheddar, destroyed
- '1 tsp cream cheddar, mollified
- 1/4 tsp preparing powder
- 1/8 tsp Italian flavoring
- 1/8 tsp garlic powder
- pinch of salt
- 3 tsp low carb marinara sauce
- 1/2 cup mozzarella cheddar
- 6 pepperonis cut down the middle
- 1 tbsp parmesan cheddar, destroyed
- 1/4 tsp basil flavoring

Directions:

1. Preheat stove to 400 degrees. Turn waffle creator on or plug it in so it gets hot.

2. In a little bowl include coconut flour, egg white, mozzarella cheddar, relaxed cream cheddar, heating powder, garlic powder, Italian seasonings, and a spot of salt.

3. Pour 1/2 of the player in the waffle producer, close the top, and cook for 3-4 minutes or until chaffle arrives at desired doneness.

4. Carefully expel chaffle from the waffle creator, at that point adhere to similar guidelines to make the second chaffle.

5. Top each chaffle with tomato sauce (I utilized 1/2 tsp per), pepperoni, mozzarella cheddar, and parmesan cheddar.

6. Place in the broiler on a preparing sheet (or straight on the heating rack) on the first-rate of the stove for 5-6 minutes. At that point turn the broiler to cook so the cheddar starts to air pocket and dark-colored. Keep a nearby eye as it can consume rapidly. I cooked my pizza chaffle for approx 1 min and 30 seconds.

7. Remove from stove and sprinkle basil on top.

436. Traditional Keto Low Carb Chaffle

Preparation time: 10 minutes
Cooking time: 5 minutes

Ingredients:

- 1 egg
- 1/2 cup cheddar, destroyed

Directions

1. Turn waffle producer on or plug it in with the goal that it warms and oil the two sides.

2. In a little bowl, split an egg at that point include the 1/2 cup cheddar and mix to consolidate.

3. Pour 1/2 of the hitter in the waffle producer and close the top.

4. Cook for 3-4 minutes or until it arrives at wanted doneness.

5. Carefully expel from waffle producer and put in a safe spot for 2-3 minutes to give it an opportunity to fresh.

6. Follow the guidelines again to make

the second chaffle.

7. This formula for a customary chaffle makes incredible sandwiches.

437. Essential Chaffle Recipe

Preparation time: 15 minutes
Cooking time: 5 minutes

Ingredients:

- 1/2 cup of cheddar, destroyed (you can utilize any cheddar)
- 1 egg
- 1 tsp of sans gluten preparing powder
- 2 tablespoons of almond flour (can substitute with 1 tablespoon of coconut flour whenever wanted)

Directions:

1. Assemble and set up the entirety of your fixings and preheat your waffle creator.
2. Combine your egg, destroyed cheddar, heating powder, and almond or coconut flour.
3. Empty a large portion of your blend into the waffle producer. Cook till done. Expel. Empty the rest of the hitter into the waffle producer and cook.
4. We purchased the little Dash brand small scale waffle producer and the lower than usual frying pan (you can utilize it is possible that one) to use with this formula and it makes the ideal size Chaffle. Try not to have a small scale waffle creator? You can utilize a standard waffle producer or skillet when necessary.

438. Lemon Delight Chaffle

Preparation time: 15 minutes
Cooking time: 0 minutes

Ingredients:

- 1 oz cream cheddar (mollified)
- 1/4 cup mozzarella cheddar, destroyed
- 1 egg
- 1 to 2 tsp lemon juice
- 2 tablespoons of sugar
- 1 tsp preparing powder
- 4 tablespoons of almond flour

Directions:

1. Add all the recipes together to get the exact formula!!!
2. Banana Nut Muffin Chaffle
3. 1 oz cream cheddar (mollified)
4. 1/4 cup mozzarella cheddar, destroyed
5. 1 egg
6. 1 tsp banana extricate
7. 2 tablespoons of sugar
8. 1 tsp preparing powder
9. 4 tablespoons of almond flour
10. 2 tablespoons of pecans or walnuts, hacked

Directions:

01. Add all the recipes together to get the exact formula!!!

439. McGriddle Chaffle

Preparation time: 15 minutes
Cooking time: 0 minutes

Ingredients:

- 1 egg
- 1 oz cream cheddar, relaxed
- 1 tsp sugar
- 1 tsp vanilla

- 1 tablespoon keto-accommodating maple syrup (We use Lakanto)
- 1/4 cup mozzarella cheddar, destroyed
- 1 tsp of heating powder
- 4 tablespoons of almond flour

Directions:

1. Add all the recipes together to get the exact formula!!!

440. Chocolate Dream Chaffle

Preparation time: 15 minutes
Cooking time: 0 minutes

Ingredients:

- 1 egg
- 1/4 cup of mozzarella cheddar
- 1 oz cream cheddar
- 2 tsp sugar
- 2 tablespoons cacao powder
- 1 tsp vanilla
- 4 Tbsp almond flour
- 1 tsp heating powder
- Red Velvet Chaffle
- 1 egg
- 1/4 cup of mozzarella cheddar
- 1 oz cream cheddar
- 2 tsp sugar
- 2 tablespoons cacao powder
- 1 tsp red velvet concentrate
- 4 Tbsp almond flour
- 1 tsp preparing powder

Directions:

1. Add all the recipes together to get the exact formula!!!

441. Keto Italian Cream Chaffle Cake

Preparation time: 15 minutes
Cooking time: 10 minutes

Ingredients:

- Sweet Chaffle Ingredients:
- 4 oz Cream Cheese relaxed and room temp
- 4 eggs
- 1 tablespoon softened margarine
- 1 teaspoon vanilla concentrate
- 1/2 teaspoon cinnamon
- 1 tablespoon monk fruit sugar or your most loved keto-endorsed sugar
- 4 tablespoons coconut flour
- 1 tablespoon almond flour
- 1 1/2 teaspoons heating powder
- 1 tbs coconut destroyed and unsweetened
- 1 tbs pecans cleaved
- Italian Cream Frosting Ingredients:
- 2 oz cream cheddar mellowed and room temp
- 2 tbs margarine room temp
- 2 tbs monk fruit sugar or your most loved keto-endorsed sugar
- 1/2 teaspoon vanilla

Directions:

1. In a medium-size blender, include the cream cheddar, eggs, softened spread, vanilla, sugar, coconut flour, almond flour, and heating powder. Discretionary: Add the destroyed coconut and pecans to the blend or spare it for the icing. Whichever way is extraordinary!

2. Blend the fixings on high until it's

smooth and rich.

3. Preheat the smaller than normal waffle creator.

4. Add the fixings to the preheated waffle creator.

5. Cook for around 2 to 3 minutes until the waffles are finished.

6. Remove and permit the chaffles to cool.

7. In a different bowl, begin to make the icing by including every one of the fixings together. Mix until it's smooth and rich.

8. Once the chaffles have totally cool, ice the cake.

9. Notes

10. Makes 8 smaller than expected chaffles or 3 to 4 huge chaffles

442. Easy Parmesan Chicken Chaffle

Preparation time: 10 minutes
Cooking time: 5 minutes

Ingredients

- Chaffle Ingredients:
- 1/2 cup canned chicken bosom
- 1/4 cup cheddar
- 1/8 cup parmesan cheddar
- 1 egg
- 1 tsp Italian flavoring
- 1/8 tsp garlic powder
- 1 tsp cream cheddar room temperature
- Besting Ingredients:
- 2 cuts of provolone cheddar
- 1 tbs sugar free pizza sauce

Directions

1. Preheat the small scale waffle creator.

2. In a medium-size bowl, include every one of the fixings and blend until it's completely joined.

3. Add a teaspoon of destroyed cheddar to the waffle iron for 30 seconds before including the blend. This will make the best outside layer and make it simpler to remove this overwhelming chaffle from the waffle creator when it's set.

4. Pour portion of the blend in the smaller than normal waffle producer and cook it for at least 4 to 5 minutes.

5. Repeat the above strides to cook the second Chicken Parmesan Chaffle.

6. Notes

7. Top with a sugar free pizza sauce and one cut of provolone cheddar. I like to sprinkle the top with much progressively Italian Seasoning as well!

443. Chickfila Copycat Chaffle Sandwich

Preparation time: 45 minutes
Cooking time: 25 minutes

Ingredients

- Elements for the Chicken:
- 1 Chicken Breast
- 4 T of Dill Pickle Juice
- 2 T Parmesan Cheese powdered
- 2 T Pork Rinds ground
- 1 T Flax Seed ground
- Salt and Pepper
- 2 T Butter dissolved
- Elements for Chaffle Sandwich Bun:
- 1 Egg room temperature

- 1 Cup Mozzarella Cheese destroyed
- 3 - 5 drops of Stevia Glycerite
- 1/4 tsp Butter Extract

Directions:

1. Directions for the Chicken:
2. Pound chicken to 1/2 inch thickness.
3. Cut down the middle and spot in zip lock baggie with pickle
4. Juice.
5. Seal baggie and spot in the cooler for 1 hour to medium-term.
6. Preheat Airfryer for 5 mins at 400
7. In a little shallow bowl, combine Parmesan cheddar, pork skins, flaxseed, and S&P.
8. Remove chicken from the baggie and dispose of pickle juice.
9. Dip chicken in dissolved margarine at that point in flavoring blend.
10. Place material paper round in Airfryer container, brush the paper daintily with oil. (I utilized coconut)
11. Place chicken in preheated Airfryer and cook for 7 minutes.
12. Flip chicken and Airfry for an extra 7-8 mins. (This can change depending on the size of your check internal temp of 165*
13. Guidelines for Chaffle Bun:
14. Mix everything in a little bowl. Put 1/4 of the blend in the preheated small scale run waffle iron. Cook for 4 mins. Expel to a cooking rack. Rehash x3
15. Assemble Sandwich's: Place laid chicken on one Chaffle bun, includes 3 dill pickle cuts. Spread with different buns. Rehash.
16. Enjoy!

444. Banana Nut Chaffle

Preparation time: 15 minutes
Cooking time: 10 minutes

Ingredients

- 1 egg
- 1 tbs cream cheddar. mellowed and room temp
- 1 tbs sugar-free cheesecake pudding discretionary fixing since it is grimy keto
- 1/2 cup mozzarella cheddar
- 1 tbs Monkfruit confectioners
- 1/4 tsp vanilla concentrate
- 1/4 tsp banana remove
- Discretionary Toppings:
- Sugar-free caramel sauce
- Pecans

Directions

1. Preheat the smaller than normal waffle producer
2. In a little bowl, whip the egg.
3. Add the rest of the fixings to the egg blend and blend it until it's very much consolidated.
4. Add a large portion of the hitter to the waffle creator and cook it for at least 4 minutes until it's brilliant dark colored.
5. Remove the completed chaffle and include the other portion of the player to cook the other chaffle.
6. Top with your discretionary fixings and serve warm!
7. Notes
8. Top with your discretionary fixings and serve warm!

445 Pumpkin Chaffle with Cream Cheese Frosting

Preparation time: 15 minutes
Cooking time: 5 minutes

Ingredients

- 1 egg
- 1/2 cup mozzarella cheddar
- 1/2 tsp pumpkin pie zest
- 1 tbs pumpkin healthy pressed with no sugar included
- Optional Cream Cheese Frosting Ingredients:
- 2 tbs cream cheddar relaxed and room temperature
- 2 tbs monk fruit confectioners mix or any of your most loved keto-accommodating sugar
- 1/2 tsp clear vanilla concentrate

Directions

1. Preheat the smaller than expected waffle creator.
2. In a little bowl, whip the egg.
3. Add the cheddar, pumpkin pie zest, and the pumpkin.
4. Mix well.
5. Add 1/2 of the blend to the smaller than expected waffle creator and cook it for in any event 3 to 4 minutes until it's brilliant dark-colored.
6. While the chaffle is cooking, include the entirety of the cream cheddar icing fixings in a bowl and blend it until it's smooth and velvety.
7. Add the cream cheddar icing to the hot chaffle and serve it right away.
8. Notes
9. Add the cream cheddar icing to the hot chaffle and serve it right away

446. Crispy Everything Bagel Chaffle Chips

Preparation time: 20 minutes
Cooking time: 5 minutes

Ingredients

- 3 Tbs Parmesan Cheese destroyed
- 1 tsp Everything Bagel Seasoning

Directions

1. Preheat the smaller than expected waffle creator.
2. Place the Parmesan cheddar on the iron and enable it to bubble. Around 3 minutes. Make sure to leave it sufficiently long or else it won't turn firm when it cools. Significant advance!
3. Sprinkle the softened cheddar with around 1 teaspoon of Everything Bagel Seasoning. Leave the waffle iron open when it cooks!
4. Unplug the scaled-down waffle producer and enable it to cool for a couple of moments. This will allow the cheddar sufficiently cool to tie together and get fresh.
5. After around 2 minutes of it chilling, it will even now be warm.
6. Use a scaled-down spatula to strip the warm (however not hot cheddar from the smaller than usual waffle iron.
7. Allow it to cool totally for fresh chips! These chips pack an incredible crunch, which is something I will in general miss on Keto!
8. Notes
9. The more cheddar you utilize, the thicker the chips will be. The less cheddar you use the lighter and increasingly fresh the chips will be! This method functions admirably for the two surfaces! Make sure to use

less Everything Bagel seasonings if you use less cheddar. You don't need the seasonings to be overwhelming to the proportion of cheddar you have

447. Keto BLT Chaffle Sandwich

Preparation time: 15 minutes
Cooking time: 5 minutes

Ingredients

- Chaffle bread fixings
- 1/2 cup mozzarella destroyed
- 1 egg
- 1 tbs green onion diced
- 1/2 tsp Italian flavoring
- Sandwich fixings
- Bacon pre-cooked
- Lettuce
- Tomato cut
- 1 tbs mayo

Directions:

1. Preheat the smaller than normal waffle creator
2. In a little bowl, whip the egg.
3. Add the cheddar, seasonings, and onion. Blend it until it's all around fused.
4. Place a large portion of the hitter in the smaller than usual waffle creator and cook it for 4 minutes.
5. If you need crunchy bread, include a tsp of destroyed cheddar to the smaller than normal waffle iron for 30 seconds before including the hitter. The additional cheddar outwardly makes the best covering!
6. After the first chaffle is finished, add the rest of the player to the smaller than usual waffle producer and cook it

for 4 minutes.

7. Add the mayo, bacon, lettuce, and tomato to your sandwich.

448. Chocolate Chip Cookie Chaffle Cake

Preparation time: 15 minutes
Cooking time: 5 minutes

Ingredients

- Elements for cake layers:
- 1 T Butter liquefied
- 1 T Golden Monkfruit sugar
- 1 Egg Yolk
- 1/8 tsp Vanilla Extract
- 1/8 tsp Cake Batter Extract
- 3 T Almond Flour
- 1/8 tsp Baking Powder
- 1 T Chocolate Chips sugar-free
- Whipped Cream Frosting Ingredients:
- 1 tsp unflavored gelatin
- 4 tsp Cold Water
- 1 Cup HWC
- 2 T Confectioners Sweetener

Directions

1. Chocolate Chip Cookie Chaffle Cake Recipe Instructions
2. Cake Instructions
3. Mix everything and cook in a smaller than normal waffle iron for 4 mins. Rehash for each layer. I decided to make 3.
4. Whipped Cream Frosting Instructions
5. Place your mixers and your blending bowl in the cooler for around 15 minutes to enable them to cool.
6. In a microwave-safe bowl, sprinkle

the gelatin over the virus water. Mix, and permit to "blossom". This takes around 5 minutes.

7. Microwave the gelatin blend for 10 seconds. It will end up being a fluid. Mix to ensure everything is broken down.

8. In your chilled blending bowl, start whipping the cream on a low speed. Include the confectioner's sugar.

9. Move to a higher speed and watch for good tops to start to the frame.

10. Once the whipping cream is beginning to top, switch back to a lower speed and gradually sprinkle the dissolved fluid gelatin blend in. When it's in, turn back to a higher speed and keep on beating until it's arrived at hardened pinnacles.

11. Place in channeling sacks and funnel on your cake.

12. Notes

13. I just utilized 1/2 of the whipped cream for this recipe.

449. Chaffle With Cranberry Purree

Preparation Time: 5 min
Cooking Time: 5 min
Servings: 4

Ingredients

- 2 large eggs
- 1/4 cup almond flour
- 3/4 tsp baking powder
- 1 cup mozzarella cheese, shredded
- Cooking spray
- ¼ cup cranberry puree cranberries for topping

Directions

1. Preheat your waffle maker according

to manufacture instructions and grease with cooking spray.

2. Crack eggs in bowl and beat with almond flour and baking powder in mixing bowl.

3. Sprinkle half of cheese batter in waffle machine and pour half of egg batter over it.

4. Close chaffle machine and cook for 2-3 minutes.

5. Once cooked remove from maker.

6. Repeat with remaining batter

7. Pour cranberry puree and cranberries over it.

8. Serve with keto coffee and enjoy!

450. Basic Chaffles Recipe For Sandwiches

Preparation Time: 5 min
Cooking Time: 5 min
Servings: 2

Ingredients

- 1/2 cup mozzarella cheese, shredded
- 1 large egg
- 2 tbsps. almond flour
- 1/2 tsp psyllium husk powder
- 1/4 tsp baking powder
- 1 tsp stevia

Directions

1. Switch on and grease your waffle maker waffle maker with cooking spray.

2. Beat egg, cheese, almond flour, husk powder and baking powder.

3. Pour batter in the middle of waffle maker and close the lid.

4. Cook chaffles for about 2-3 minutes until cooked and light brown in color.

5. Carefully transfer chaffles to plate.

6. Serve with strawberry slice.

7. Enjoy!

451. Savory Garlic Parmesan Chaffles

Preparation Time: 5 min
Cooking Time: 5 min
Servings: 4

Ingredients

- 1/2 cup cheddar cheese, shredded
- 1/3 cup parmesan cheese
- 1 large egg
- ½ tbsp. garlic powder
- 1/2 tsp onion powder
- 1/4 tsp baking powder
- 1 pinch salt

Directions

1. Switch on your waffle maker and lightly grease your waffle maker with cooking spray.

2. Beat egg with garlic powder, onion powder, salt and baking powder in small mixing bowl.

3. Sprinkle ½ both cheese on waffle maker

4. Pour half of the egg batter into the middle of your waffle iron and close the lid.

5. Cook chaffles for about 2-3 minutes until crispy.

6. Once cooked remove chaffles from maker.

7. Drizzle garlic powder on top and enjoy!

452. Almond Flour Chaffles

Preparation Time: 5 min
Cooking Time: 5 min
Servings: 2

Ingredients

- 1 large egg
- 3/4 cup cheddar cheese, shredded
- 2 tbsps. almond flour
- 2 tbsps. cream cheese
- 1 tsp. stevia
- 1/2 tsp cinnamon powder
- 1/2 tsp vanilla extract
- 1/2 tsp psyllium husk powder
- 1/4 tsp baking powder

Directions

1. Switch on your waffle maker.

2. Grease your waffle maker with cooking spray and heat up on medium.

3. In a mixing bowl, beat egg with coconut flour, oil, stevia, cinnamon powder, vanilla, husk powder and baking powder.

4. Once egg is beaten well, add in cheese and mix again.

5. Pour half of the waffle batter into the middle of your waffle iron and close the lid.

6. Cook chaffles for about 2-3 minutes until crispy.

7. Serve with keto hot chocolate and enjoy!

453. Pumpkin Chaffles with Strawberries

Preparation Time: 5 min
Cooking Time: 5 min

Servings: 2

Ingredients

- 1/2 oz. cream cheese
- 1 large egg
- 1/2 cup mozzarella cheese, shredded
- 1 tsp. stevia
- 3 tsps. almond flour
- 1/2 tbsps. pumpkin pie spice
- 1/2 tsp vanilla extract
- 1/4 tsp baking powder

Directions

1. Grease your Belgian waffle maker with cooking spray and switch on.
2. Crack eggs in mixing bowl and with coconut flour, pumpkin spice, stevia, pumpkin spice, vanilla extract and baking powder.
3. Once ingredients are mix together with egg add in cheese and mix again.
4. Pour half of the chaffles batter into the middle of your waffle iron and close the lid.
5. Cook chaffles for about 2-3 until cooked and light golden.
6. Repeat with remaining batter
7. Once chaffles are cooked remove from maker.
8. Serve with BLT coffee and enjoy!

454. Spicy Jalapeno & Tomato Chaffle

Preparation Time: 5 min
Cooking Time: 5 min
Servings: 2

Ingredients

- 1 oz. cream cheese
- 1 large egg

- 1 pinch salt
- 1/2 cup cheddar cheese
- 1 tomato chopped
- 1 jalapenos chopped
- 1/4 tsp baking powder

Directions

1. Switch on your waffle maker and grease with cooking spray and let it preheat.
2. Beat egg with salt, baking powder and cream cheese in bowl.
3. Sprinkle chop tomato, jalapeno and cheese in waffle maker.
4. Pour egg mixture over cheese, close waffle maker.
5. Cook the chaffles for about 2-3 minutes until brown.
6. Once chaffles are cooked remove from maker.
7. Serve hot and enjoy!

455. Strawberries Purre Chaffles

Preparation Time: 5 min
Cooking Time: 5 min
Servings: 2

Ingredients

- 1 egg
- 1 cup mozzarella cheese, shredded
- 1 tbsp. almond flour
- 1/4 cup strawberry puree
- 1 tbsp. coconut flour for topping
- Berries for topping

Directions

1. Preheat your waffle maker as per the manufacturer instructions.
2. Grease your waffle maker with

coconut oil.

3. Mix together egg, almond flour, and strawberry purée.

4. Add cheese and mix until well combined.

5. Pour batter in preheated and greased waffle maker and close the lid.

6. Cook strawberry chaffles for about 3-4 minutes or until cooked through.

7. Once cooked remove from maker

8. Drizzle coconut flour and berries on top.

9. Enjoy!

456. Simple Keto Cocoa Chaffles

Preparation Time: 5 min
Cooking Time: 5 min
Servings: 2

Ingredients

- 1 large egg
- 1/2 cup shredded mozzarella cheese
- 1 tbsp. cocoa powder
- 2 tbsps. almond flour

Directions

1. Preheat your round waffle maker on medium high heat.

2. Mix together egg, cheese, almond flour, cocoa powder and vanilla in small mixing bowl.

3. Pour chaffles mixture into the center of the waffle iron.

4. Close the waffle maker and let cook for 3-5 minutes or until waffle is golden brown and set.

5. Carefully remove chaffles from the waffle maker.

6. Serve hot and enjoy!

457. Simple Crispy Coconut Chaffle

Preparation Time: 5 min
ooking Time: 5 min
Servings: 2

Ingredients

- 1 large egg
- 1/2 cup shredded mozzarella cheese
- 2 tbsps. coconut flour

Directions

1. Preheat your square waffle maker on medium high heat.

2. Mix together egg, cheese and coconut flour in bowl.

3. Pour coconut chaffle batter in greased waffle maker.

4. Cook chaffles for 2-3 minutes or until cooked.

5. Once chaffle are cooked carefully removed from make.

6. Drizzle coconut flour and keto melted chocolate over it.

7. Serve hot and enjoy!

458. Morning Ham Chaffles Sandwich

Preparation Time: 5 min
Cooking Time: 5 min
Servings: 4

Ingredients

- 1 cup egg whites
- 1 cup cheddar cheese shredded
- ¼ cup almond flour
- ¼ cup heavy cream
- Topping
- 2 tomatoes, slice
- 4 ham slice

- 1 cucumber, sliced
- 1 scramble egg

Directions

1. Preheat your square waffle maker and grease with cooking spray.
2. Beat egg white in small bowl with flour.
3. Add shredded cheese in egg whites and mix well.
4. Add cream and cheese in egg mixture.
5. Pour Chaffles batter in waffle maker and close the lid.
6. Cook chaffles for about 4 minutes until crispy and brown.
7. Carefully remove chaffles from maker.
8. Serve with ham slice, scramble egg, tomato slice, cucumber slice.
01. Enjoy!

459. Brunch Chaffle Bowl

Preparation Time: 5 min
Cooking Time: 10 min
Srvings: 2

Ingredients

- 1/2 cup cheddar cheese
- 1/2 tsp. baking powder
- 1/4 cup egg whites
- Serving
- 1 egg fried
- 4 slice bacon
- salt and pepper to taste
- 1 tsp. avocado oil
- Berries for topping
- Keto chocolate sauce

Directions

1. Mix together all ingredients in a bowl.
2. Allow batter to sit while waffle iron warms.
3. Spray waffle iron with nonstick cooking spray.
4. Pour batter in waffle maker and cook according to directions of manufacturer.
5. Meanwhile heat oil in pan and fry bacon for 4-5 minutes until crispy. transfer cooked bacon in another plate.
6. Fry egg in same pan according to your choice.
7. Serve chaffles with berries, bacon, chocolate sauce and fried egg.
8. Enjoy!

460. Bacon Chaffles With Egg & Asparagus

Preparation Time: 5 min
Cooking Time: 10 min
Servings: 1

Ingredients

- 1 egg
- 1/4 cup cheddar cheese
- 2 tbsps. almond flour
- ½ tsp. baking powder
- 1 bacon slice, cooked
- TOPPING
- 1 egg
- 4-5 stalks asparagus
- 1 tsp avocado oil

Directions

1. Preheat waffle maker to medium high heat.
2. Mix chaffle ingredients in bowl except

bacon.

3. Sprinkle cooked chopped bacon slice over waffle maker.

4. Spoon chaffles batter into the center of the waffle iron and cook for 2-3 minutes.

5. Meanwhile Sautee asparagus in heated oil and poach egg in boil water.

6. Once Chaffles are cooked remove from maker.

7. Serve chaffles with poach egg and asparagus

461. Coconut Chaffles With Boil Egg

Preparation Time: 5 min
Cooking Time: 5 min
Servings: 2

Ingredients

- 1 egg
- 1 oz. cream cheese,
- 1 oz. cheddar cheese
- 2 tbsps. coconut flour
- 1 tsp. stevia
- 1 egg, soft boil for serving

Directions

1. Heat you mini Dash waffle maker and grease with cooking spray.

2. Mix together all chaffles ingredients in bowl.

3. Pour chaffle batter in preheated waffle maker.

4. Close the lid.

5. Cook chaffles for about 2-3 minutes until golden brown.

6. Serve with boil egg an enjoy!

462. Chaffle With Parmeson

Preparation Time: 5 min
Cooking Time: 10 min
Servings: 1

Ingredients

- 1 egg
- 1/4 cup shredded cheddar cheese
- 2 tbsps. almond flour
- 1 tsp Italian seasoning
- ¼ cup parmesan cheese for topping

Directions

1. Mix together egg cheese, almond flour and seasoning in bowl.

2. Switch on and grease waffle maker with cooking spray.

3. Pour batter in preheated waffle maker.

4. Cook chaffles for about 2-3 minutes until the chaffle is cooked through.

5. Meanwhile fry egg in non-stick pan for about 1-2 minutes.

6. For serving set fried egg on chaffles with feta cheese and tomatoes slice

463. Chaffle With Herbs

Preparation Time: 10 min
Cooking Time: 5 min
Servings: 1

Ingredients

- 1 large egg
- 1/4 cup cheddar cheese, shredded
- 1 tbsp. almond flour
- ¼ tsp. baking powder
- ½ tsp. garlic powder
- 1 tbsp. minced parsley
- For Serving

- 1 poach egg
- 4 oz. smoked salmon

Directions

1. Preheat your dash mini waffle maker and let it heat up and grease with cooking spray.

2. Mix together egg, cheese, almond flour, baking powder, garlic powder, parsley to a mixing bowl until combined well.

3. Pour batter in dash mini waffle maker.

4. Close the lid.

5. Cook chaffles for about 2-3 minutes or until cooked or no soggy.

6. Serve chaffles in plate with smoked salmon and poach egg.

01. Enjoy!

464. Chaffle Taco With Raspberries

Preparation Time: 5 min
Cooking Time: 15 min
Servings: 1

Ingredients

- 1 egg
- 1/4 cup mozzarella cheese, shredded
- 1/4 cup cheddar cheese, shredded
- 1 tsp coconut flour
- 1/4 tsp baking powder
- 1/2 tsp stevia
- For Topping
- 4 oz. raspberries
- 2 tbsps. coconut flour
- 2 oz. raspberry puree

Directions

1. Switch on your round waffle maker and grease is with cooking spray.

2. Mix together all chaffle ingredients in bowl and beat with fork.

3. Cook round chaffle in greased chaffle maker.

4. Once cooked remove from maker and immediately roll over kitchen roller for 5 minutes.

5. Meanwhile coat raspberries with in sauce and set on chaffle taco.

6. Sprinkle coconut flour on top.

7. Enjoy chaffle taco as dessert!

465. Chaffle Sandwich With Chicken

Preparation Time: 5 min
Cooking Time: 15 min
Servings: 2

Ingredients

- 1 large egg
- 1 cup cheddar cheese, shredded
- 1 pinch salt
- 1 tsp. baking powder
- For Serving
- 1 chicken thigh
- salt
- pepper
- 1 tsp. garlic, minced
- I tsp avocado oil
- 1 cucumber sliced
- 4-5 lettuce leaves
- 1 tomato sliced
- 4 slice cheddar cheese.

Directions

1. Heat Belgian waffle maker and grease with cooking spray.

2. Mix together chaffle ingredients and make two Belgian chaffles batter in

skillet and cook for about 2-3 minutes.

3. Meanwhile heat oil in pan, over medium heat.

4. Coat chicken thigh with salt, pepper and garlic.

5. Cook coated thigh in oil for about 4-5 minutes until cooked through.

6. Transfer cooked on Belgian chaffle top with lettuce leaves, tomato slice, cucumber slice, and lettuce leaves.

7. Cover sandwich and drizzle flax seeds on top.

8. Serve and enjoy!

466. Nutritious Creamy Chaffles

Preparation time: 5 min
Cooking time: 4 min
Servings: 2

Ingredients

- Eggs – 2
- Mozzarella – 1 cup
- Cream cheese – 2 tablespoons
- Almond flour – 2 tablespoons
- Baking powder – ¾ tablespoons
- Water (optional) – 2 tablespoons

Directions

1. Pre-heat waffle iron

2. Put listed ingredients in some bowl and mix

3. Grease waffle iron slightly and cook the mixture in it till crisp

467. Crunchy Jalapeno Chaffles

Preparation time: 4 min
Cooking time: 4 min
Servings: 2

Ingredients

- Eggs – 2
- Cheddar cheese – 1 ½ cups
- Jalapeno pepper – 16 slices

Directions:

1. Preheat waffle maker

2. Mix eggs and ¾ cups of cheddar cheese in a bowl

3. Shred cheddar cheese on waffle maker plate

4. Pour mixture onto plate

5. Add cheese on top of mixture

6. Top up with 4 Jalapeno slices and cook till crunchy

468. Crispy Simple Chaffles

Preparation time: 5 min
Cooking time: 10 min
Servings: 2

Ingredients

- Cheddar cheese (shredded) – 1/3 cup
- Eggs – 1
- Baking powder – ¼ teaspoon
- Flaxseed (ground) – 1 teaspoon
- Parmesan cheese (shredded) – 1/3 cup

Directions:

1. Mix all ingredients except parmesan cheese in one bowl

2. Shred half parmesan cheese on waffle iron to grease plate

3. Pour mixture and top with remaining shredded parmesan cheese

4. Cook till crispy

469. Bacon Bite Chaffles

Preparation time: 5 min

Cooking time: 5 min
Servings: 2

Ingredients

- Bacon bites (as desired)
- Cheddar cheese – 1 ½ cups

Directions:

1. Pre-heat waffle iron
2. Mix all ingredients in one bowl
3. Lightly grease waffle iron
4. Pour mixture and cook till crisp

470. Eggplant Chaffles

Preparation time: 10 min
Cooking time: 10 min
Servings: 2

Ingredients

- Eggplant – 1 medium
- Eggs – 1
- (Cheddar cheese – 1 ½ cups

Directions:

1. Boil eggplant for 15 min then blend
2. Preheat waffle iron
3. Mix listed ingredients in one bowl
4. Grease waffle iron, pour mixture and cook till crisp

471. Bacon Cheese Chaffles

Preparation time: 10 min

Cooking time: 10 min

Servings: 2

Ingredients

- Swiss cheese (shredded) – ½ cup
- Jalapenos (diced)– 1
- Bacon pieces – 2

- Eggs – 1

Directions:

1. Pre-heat waffle iron and grease
2. Fry bacon pieces in a pan
3. Add shredded cheese, egg and jalapenos and mix together
4. Cook till crisp

472. Crunchy Bacon Chaffles

Preparation time: 5 min
Cooking time: 5 min
Servings: 2

Ingredients

- Cheddar – 1/3 cup
- Eggs – 1
- Flaxseed (ground) – 1 teaspoon
- Baking powder – ¼ teaspoon
- Bacon piece – 2 tablespoons
- Parmesan – 1/3 cup

Directions:

1. Cook bacon in pan
2. Add egg, cheddar cheese, flaxseed and baking powder then mix
3. Shred part of parmesan cheese in waffle iron and grease plate
4. Pour mixture and top with remaining parmesan cheese
5. Cook till crisp

473. Crunchy Pickle Chaffles

Preparation time: 5 min
Cooking time: 5 min
Servings: 2

Ingredients

- Mozzarella – ½ cup

231

- Eggs – 1
- Pork Panko bread crumbs – ½ cup
- Pickle juice – 1 tablespoon
- Pickle slices – 8

Directions:

1. Pre-heat waffle iron
2. Mix ingredients together and pour thin layer onto waffle iron
3. Add drained pickle slices
4. Top with remaining mixture and cook till crisp

474. Olive Chaffles

Preparation time: 5 min
Cooking time: 5 min
Servings: 2

Ingredients

- Cheddar – 1/3 cup
- Parmesan – 1/3 cup
- Eggs – 1
- Baking powder – ¼ teaspoon
- Flaxseed (ground) – 1 teaspoon
- Olive (sliced) – 6 to 8
- Several sun-dried tomatoes

Directions:

1. Add cheddar cheese, flaxseed, egg and baking powder in a bowl and mix
2. Chop the tomatoes finely and add them to the mix.
3. Shred half parmesan cheese on waffle iron and lightly grease plate
4. Pour mixture and top with olives and remaining parmesan cheese
5. Cook till crisp
6. Takes 5 min to prepare and serves 2

475. Halloumi Chaffles

Preparation time: 5 min
Cooking time: 6 min
Servings: 2

Ingredients

- Pasta sauce – 2 tablespoons
- Halloumi – 3 oz

Directions:

1. Cut halloumi cheese into half inch slices
2. Place cheese in waffle maker then turn on
3. Cook for about 6 min till golden brown
4. Spread sauce on chaffle

476. Chickfila Chaffles

Preparation time: 20 min
Cooking time: 5 min
Servings: 2

Ingredients

- For chicken
- Chicken breast pieces – 1
- Pickle juice – 4 tablespoons
- Parmesan – 4 tablespoons
- Pork rinds – 2 tablespoons
- Butter – 1 teaspoon
- Flaxseed (ground) – 1 teaspoon
- Salt (as desired)
- Black pepper powder – ¼ teaspoon
- For bun
- Shredded mozzarella – 1 cup
- Egg – 1
- Butter extract – ¼ teaspoon

- Stevia glycerite – 4 drops

Directions:

1. Cut half- inch chicken pieces and soak in pickle juice for one hour minimum
2. Pre-heat air fryer
3. Mix all other chicken ingredients in one bowl
4. Drain pickle juice and add chicken into bowl
5. Let chicken cook for 6 min on each side at 400°
6. Mix all bun ingredients together in one bowl
7. Place in waffle maker to cook for about 4 min
8. Sandwich the cooked chicken between the buns

477. Bacon and Egg Chaffles

Preparation time: 5 min

Cooking time: 5 min

Servings: 2

Ingredients

- For Chaffles
- Cheddar – 1 cup
- Eggs – 2
- For Sandwich
- American cheese – 2 slices
- Bacon pieces – 4
- Eggs – 2

Directions:

1. Pre-heat and grease waffle maker
2. Mix eggs and cheddar cheese together
3. Pour mixture onto waffle plate and cook till crunchy

4. Cook bacon pieces till crispy then dry then
5. Fry eggs and add them in between two chaffles alongside bacon and cheese slices

478. Almond Sandwich Chaffles

Preparation time: 5 min

Cooking time: 5 min

Servings: 2

Ingredients

- Cheddar cheese (shredded) – 1 cup
- Eggs – 2
- Almond flour – 2 tablespoons

Directions:

1. Pre-heat and grease waffle iron
2. Mix cheddar cheese and eggs in one bowl
3. Add the almond flour into mixture to enhance texture
4. Pour mixture onto waffle plate and cook till crunchy
5. Garnish ready and slightly cooled chaffles with preferred garnish
6. Takes 5 min to prepare and serves 2

479. BLT Chaffles

Preparation time: 5 min

Cooking time: 5 min

Servings: 2

Ingredients

Mozzarella cheese (shredded) – 1 cup

Eggs – 2

Green onion (diced) – 1 tbsp

Italian seasoning – ½ teaspoon

For Sandwich

Bacon – 4 strips

Tomato (sliced) - 1

Green Lettuce – 2 leaves

Mayo – 2 tablespoons

Directions:

1. Pre-heat and grease waffle maker

2. Mix all ingredients in one bowl

3. Pour mixture onto waffle plate and spread evenly

4. Cook till crunchy then leave to cool for a minute

5. Serve with lettuce, tomato and mayo

480. Katsu Chaffles

Preparation time: 10 min
Cooking time: 5 min
Servings: 2

Ingredients

- Mozzarella cheese (shredded) – 1 cup
- Eggs – 2
- Lettuce (optional) – 2 leaves
- For sauce
- Ketchup (sugar free) – 2 tablespoons
- Oyster sauce – 1 tablespoon
- Worcestershire/Worcester sauce – 2 tablespoons
- Monk fruit/swerve – 1 teaspoon
- For chicken
- Chicken thigh (boneless) – 2 pieces
- Almond flour – 1 cup
- Salt (as desired)
- Eggs – 1
- Black pepper – (as desired)
- Vegetable cooking oil – 2 cups

- Pork rinds – 3 oz
- Brine
- Salt – 1 tablespoon
- Water – 2 cups

Directions:

1. Boil chicken for 30 min then pat it dry

2. Add black pepper and salt to the chicken

3. Mix oyster sauce, Worcestershire sauce , ketchup and Swerve/Monkfruit in one bowl then set aside

4. Grind pork rinds into fine crumbs

5. In separate bowls, add the almond flour, beaten eggs and the crushed pork then coat your chicken pieces using these ingredients in their listed order

6. Fry coated chicken till golden brown

7. Pre-heat and grease waffle maker

8. Mix eggs and mozzarella cheese together in a bowl

9. Pour into waffle maker and cook till crunchy

10. Wash and dry green lettuces

11. Spread previously prepared sauces on one chaffle, place some lettuce, one chicken katsu then add one more chaffle

481. Veggie Sandwich Chaffles

Preparation time: 10 min
Cooking time: 5 min

Ingredients

- Mozzarella cheese (shredded) – 1 cup
- Eggs – 2
- For vegetables

- Tomato (sliced) – 1 small
- Onion (sliced) – 1 small
- Cauliflower – 1 cup
- Black pepper (as desired)
- Salt (as desired)
- For sauce
- Oyster sauce – 1 tablespoon
- Ketchup – 2 tablespoons
- Monk fruit/swerve – 1 teaspoon
- Worcestershire sauce – 2 tablespoons

Directions:

1. Mix ketchup, Swerve/Monk fruit, Worcestershire sauce and oyster sauce in a bowl
2. Boil cauliflower, strain excess water then add pepper and salt for taste
3. Pre-heat and grease waffle maker
4. Mix eggs and chaffle ingredients in one bowl
5. Pour mixture onto waffle plate and spread evenly and cook till crunchy
6. Allow the chaffles to cool for a minute then serve with already prepared vegetables and sauce

482. Cinnamon Maple Chaffles

Preparation time: 10 min
Cooking time: 5 min

Ingredients

- Mozzarella (shredded) – ½ cup
- Egg – 1
- Low carb maple syrup – 1 tablespoon
- Baking powder – ½ teaspoon
- Quinoa flour – 1 tablespoon
- Cinnamon – a sprinkle

Directions:

1. Mix all the ingredients properly and then cook in waffle maker till crispy.

483. Nutmeg Swirl Chaffles

Preparation time: 10 min
Cooking time: 5 min
Servings:

Ingredients

- Provolone cheese shredded – 1 oz
- Egg – 1
- Vanilla extract – 1 teaspoon
- Coconut flour – 1 teaspoon
- Nutmeg – 1 teaspoon
- Cinnamon – ½ teaspoon
- Sweetener (of your choice) – 1 tablespoon
- Icing
- Cream cheese (softened) – 1 oz
- Unsalted butter – 1 tablespoon
- Sweetener of your preference (low carb) – 1 tablespoon
- Vanilla – ½ teaspoon

Directions:

1. Mix ingredients for chaffles pour this mixture onto waffle plate and spread evenly and cook till crunchy.
2. Mix ingredients for the icing and sprinkle it over your chaffles.
3. Enjoy!

484. Carrot Chaffle Cake

Preparation Time: 15 minutes
Cooking Time: 24 minutes
Servings: 6

Ingredients:

- 1 egg, beaten
- 2 tablespoons melted butter
- ½ cup carrot, shredded
- ¾ cup almond flour
- 1 teaspoon baking powder
- 2 tablespoons heavy whipping cream
- 2 tablespoons sweetener
- 1 tablespoon walnuts, chopped
- 1 teaspoon pumpkin spice
- 2 teaspoons cinnamon

Directions:

1. Preheat your waffle maker.
2. In a large bowl, combine all the ingredients.
3. Pour some of the mixture into the waffle maker.
4. Close and cook for 4 minutes.

Repeat steps until all the remaining batter has been used.

485. Cereal Chaffle Cake

Preparation Time: 5 minutes
Cooking Time: 8 minutes
Servings: 2

Ingredients:

- 1 egg
- 2 tablespoons almond flour
- ½ teaspoon coconut flour
- 1 tablespoon melted butter
- 1 tablespoon cream cheese
- 1 tablespoon plain cereal, crushed
- ¼ teaspoon vanilla extract
- ¼ teaspoon baking powder
- 1 tablespoon sweetener

- 1/8 teaspoon xanthan gum

Directions:

1. Plug in your waffle maker to preheat.
2. Add all the ingredients in a large bowl.
3. Mix until well blended.
4. Let the batter rest for 2 minutes before cooking.
5. Pour half of the mixture into the waffle maker.
6. Seal and cook for 4 minutes.
7. Make the next chaffle using the same steps.

486. Easy Soft Cinnamon Rolls Chaffle Cake

Preparation time: 5 minutes
Cooking time: 12 minutes
Servings: 3

Ingredients

- 1 egg
- 1/2 cup mozzarella cheese
- 1/2 tsp vanilla
- 1/2 tsp cinnamon
- 1 tbs monk fruit confectioners blend

Directions:

1. Put the eggs in a small bowl.
2. Add the remaining ingredients.
3. Spray to the waffle maker with a non-stick cooking spray.
4. Make two chaffles.
5. Separate the mixture.
6. Cook half of the mixture for about 4 minutes or until golden.
7. Notes Added Glaze: 1 tb of cream cheese melted in a microwave for 15 seconds, and 1 tb of monk fruit

confectioners mix. Mix it and spread it over the moist fabric.

8. Additional Frosting: 1 tb cream cheese (high temp), 1 tb room temp butter (low temp) and 1 tb mmonk fruit confectioners' mix. Mix all the ingredients together and spread to the top of the cloth.

9. Top with optional frosting, glaze, nuts, sugar-free syrup, whipped cream or simply dust with monk fruit sweets.

487. Banana Pudding Chaffle Cake

Preparation time: 5 minutes
Cooking time: 5 minutes
Servings: 2

Ingredients

- 1 large egg yolk
- 1/2 cup fresh cream
- 3 T powder sweetener
- 1 / 4-1 / 2 teaspoon xanthan gum
- 1/2 teaspoon banana extract
- Banana chaffle ingredients
- 1 oz softened cream cheese
- 1/4 cup mozzarella cheese shredded
- 1 egg
- 1 teaspoon banana extract
- 2 T sweetener
- 1 tsp baking powder
- 4 T almond flour

Directions:

1. Mix heavy cream, powdered sweetener and egg yolk in a small pot. Whisk constantly until the sweetener has dissolved and the mixture is thick.

2. Cook for 1 minute. Add xanthan gum and whisk.

3. Remove from heat, add a pinch of salt

and banana extract and stir well.

4. Transfer to a glass dish and cover the pudding with plastic wrap. Refrigerate.

5. Mix all ingredients together. Cook in a preheated mini waffle maker.

488. Keto Peanut Butter Chaffle Cake

Preparation time: 5 minutes
Cooking time: 5 minutes
Servings: 2

Ingredients

- Ingredients for peanut butter chaffle:
- 2 Tbs Sugar Free Peanut Butter Powder
- 2 Tbs Monkfruit Confectioner's
- 1 egg
- 1/4 teaspoon baking powder
- 1 Tbs Heavy Whipped Cream
- 1/4 teaspoon peanut butter extract
- Peanut butter frosting ingredients
- 2 Tbs Monkfruit Confectioners
- 1 Tbs butter softens, room temperature
- 1 tbs unsweetened natural peanut butter or peanut butter powder
- 2 Tbs cream cheese softens, room temperature
- 1/4 tsp vanilla

Directions:

1. Serve the eggs in a small bowl.

2. Add the remaining ingredients and mix well until the dough is smooth and creamy.

3. If you don't have peanut butter extract, you can skip it. It adds

absolutely wonderful, more powerful peanut butter flavor and is worth investing in this extract.

4. Pour half of the butter into a mini waffle maker and cook for 2-3 minutes until it is completely cooked.

5. In another small bowl, add sweetener, cream cheese, sugar-free natural peanut butter and vanilla. Mix frosting until everything is well incorporated.

6. When the waffle cake has completely cooled to room temperature, spread the frosting.

7. Or you can even pipe the frost!

8. Or you can heat the frosting and add 1/2 teaspoon of water to make the peanut butter aze pill and drizzle over the peanut butter chaffle! I like it anyway!

489. Jicama Loaded Baked Potato Chaffle

Preparation time: 10 minutes
Cooking time: 10 minutes
Servings: 4

Ingredients:

- 1 large jicama root
- 1/2 medium onion minced
- 2 garlic cloves pressed
- 1 cup cheese of choice
- 2 eggs whisked
- Salt and Pepper

Directions:

1. Peel jicama and shred in food processor

2. Place shredded jicama in a large colander, sprinkle with 1-2 tsp of salt. Mix well and allow to drain.

3. Squeeze out as much liquid as possible (very important step)

4. Microwave for 5-8 minutes

5. Mix all ingredients together

6. Sprinkle a little cheese on waffle iron before adding 3 T of the mixture, sprinkle a little more cheese on top of the mixture

7. Cook for 5 minutes. Flip and cook 2 more.

8. Top with a dollop of sour cream, bacon pieces, cheese, and chives!

490. German Chocolate Chaffle Cake Recipe

Preparation time: 30 minutes
Cooking time: 15 minutes
Servings: 4

Ingredients:

- 2 eggs
- 1 tablespoon melted butter
- 1 tablespoon cream cheese softened to room temperature
- 2 tablespoons unsweetened cocoa powder or unsweetened raw cacao powder
- 2 tablespoons almond flour
- 2 teaspoons coconut flour
- 2 tablespoons Pyure granulated sweetener blend
- 1/2 teaspoon baking powder
- 1/2 teaspoon instant coffee granules dissolved in 1 tablespoon hot water
- 1/2 teaspoon vanilla extract
- 2 pinches salt
- German Chocolate Chaffle Cake Filling Ingredients:
- 1 egg yolk

- 1/4 cup heavy cream
- 2 tablespoons Pyure granulated sweetener blend
- 1 tablespoon butter
- 1/2 teaspoon caramel or maple extract
- 1/4 cup chopped pecans
- 1/4 cup unsweetened flaked coconut
- 1 teaspoon coconut flour

Directions:

1. Chaffle Instructions:
2. Preheat mini Dash waffle iron until thoroughly hot.
3. In a medium bowl, whisk all ingredients together until well combined.
4. Spoon a heaping 2 tablespoons of batter into waffle iron, close and cook 3-5 minutes, until done.
5. Remove to a wire rack.
6. Repeat 3 times.
7. Filling Instructions:
8. In a small saucepan over medium heat, combine the egg yolk, heavy cream, butter, and sweetener.
9. Simmer slowly, constantly stirring for 5 minutes.
10. Remove from heat and stir in extract, pecans, flaked coconut, and coconut flour.
11. Assembly:
12. Spread one-third of the filling in between each of 2 layers of chaffles and the remaining third on top chaffle and serve.

491. Keto Boston cream pie Chaffle Cake Recipe

Preparation time: 30 minutes

Cooking time: 15 minutes
Servings: 4
Ingredients:

- Chaffle Cake Ingredients:
- 2 eggs
- 1/4 cup almond flour
- 1 tsp coconut flour
- 2 tbsp melted butter
- 2 tbsp cream cheese room temp
- 20 drops Boston Cream extract
- 1/2 tsp vanilla extract
- 1/2 tsp baking powder
- 2 tbsp swerve confectioner's sweetener or monk fruit
- 1/4 tsp Xanthan powder
- Custard Ingredients:
- 1/2 cup heavy whipping cream
- 1/2 tsp Vanilla extract
- 1 /2 tbs Swerve confectioners Sweetener
- 2 Egg Yolks
- 1/8 tsp Xanthan Gum
- Ganache Ingredients:
- 2 tbs heavy whipping cream
- 2 tbs Unsweetened Baking chocolate bar chopped
- 1 tbs Swerve Confectioners Sweetener

Directions:

1. Preheat the mini waffle iron to make cake chaffles first.
2. In a blender, combine all the cake ingredients and blend it on high until it's smooth and creamy. This should only take a couple of minutes.
3. On the stovetop, heat the heavy whipping cream to a boil. While it's

heating, whisk the egg yolks and Swerve together in a separate small bowl.

4. Once the cream is boiling, pour half of it into the egg yolks. Make sure you are whisking it together while you pour in the mixture slowly.

5. Pour the egg and cream mixture back into the stovetop pan into the rest of the cream and stir continuously for another 2-3 minutes.

6. Take the custard off the heat and whisk in your vanilla & xanthan gum. Then set it aside to cool and thicken.

7. Put ingredients for the ganache in a small bowl. Microwave for 20 seconds, stir. Repeat if needed. Careful not to overheat the ganache and burn it. Only do 20 seconds at a time until it's fully melted.

8. Serve your Boston cream pie Chaffle Cake and Enjoy!!

492. Almond Joy Cake Chaffle Recipe

Preparation time: 30 minutes
Cooking time: 15 minutes
Servings: 6

Ingredients:

- Chocolate Chaffles:
- 1 egg
- 1 ounce cream cheese
- 1 tablespoon almond flour
- 1 tablespoon unsweetened cocoa powder
- 1 tablespoon erythritol sweeteners blends such as Swerve, Pyure or Lakanto
- 1/2 teaspoon vanilla extract
- 1/4 teaspoon instant coffee powder

- Coconut Filling:
- 1 1/2 teaspoons coconut oil melted
- 1 tablespoon heavy cream
- 1/4 cup unsweetened finely shredded coconut
- 2 ounces cream cheese
- 1 tablespoon confectioner's sweetener such as Swerve
- 1/4 teaspoon vanilla extract
- 14 whole almonds

Directions:

1. For the Chaffles:

2. Preheat mini Dash waffle iron until thoroughly hot.

3. In a medium bowl, whisk all chaffle ingredients together until well combined.

4. Pour half of the batter into the waffle iron.

5. Close and cook 3-5 minutes, until done. Remove to a wire rack.

6. Repeat for the second chaffle.

7. For the Filling:

8. Soften cream to room temperature or warm in the microwave for 10 seconds.

9. Add all ingredients to a bowl and mix until smooth and well-combined.

10. Assembly:

11. Spread half the filling on one chaffle and place 7 almonds evenly on top of the filling.

12. Repeat with the second chaffle and stack together.

493. Protein Vanilla Chaffle Sticks

Preparation time: 10 minutes
Cooking time: 28 minutes

Servings: 4

Ingredients:

- ½ scoop zero-carb protein powder
- 1 cup finely grated mozzarella cheese
- 2 eggs, beaten
- 1 tbsp erythritol
- ½ tsp vanilla extract

Directions:

1. Preheat the waffle iron.
2. In a medium bowl, mix the protein powder, mozzarella cheese, eggs, erythritol, and vanilla extract until well combined.
3. Open the iron and pour in a quarter of the batter. Close the iron and cook until golden brown and crispy, 7 minutes.
4. Remove the chaffle onto a plate and set aside.
5. Make three more chaffles after and transfer to a plate to cool.
01. Before enjoying, slice each chaffle into 4 sticks and serve.

494. Keto Oreo Chaffles

Preparation time: 13 minutes
Cooking time: 28 minutes
Servings: 4

- **Ingredients:**
- For the Oreo chaffles:
- 2 eggs, beaten
- 1 cup finely grated mozzarella cheese
- 2 tbsp almond flour
- 1 tbsp unsweetened dark cocoa powder
- 2 tbsp erythritol
- 1 tbsp cream cheese, softened

- ½ tsp vanilla extract
- For the glaze:
- 1 tbsp swerve confectioner's sugar
- 1 tsp water

Directions:

1. Preheat the waffle iron.
2. In a medium bowl, combine all the ingredients for the Oreo chaffles until adequately mixed.
3. Open the iron and pour in a quarter of the batter. Close the iron and cook until crispy, 7 minutes.
4. Remove the chaffle onto a plate and set aside.
5. Make 3 more chaffles with the remaining batter and transfer to a plate to cool.
6. For the glaze:
7. In a small bowl, whisk the swerve confectioner's sugar and water until smooth.
8. Drizzle a little of the glaze over each chaffle and serve after.

495. Keto Chaffle Churro Sticks

Preparation time: 10 minutes
Cooking time: 28 minutes
Servings: 4

Ingredients:

- 1 egg, beaten
- ½ cup finely grated mozzarella cheese
- 2 tbsp swerve brown sugar
- ½ tsp cinnamon powder

Directions:

1. Preheat the waffle iron.
2. Combine all the ingredients in a medium bowl until smooth.

3. Open the iron and pour in a quarter of the mixture. Close the iron and cook until golden brown and crispy, 7 minutes.

4. Remove the chaffle onto a plate and set aside.

5. Make 3 more chaffles with the remaining ingredients

6. Cut the chaffles into 4 sticks and serve after.

496. Chocolate Chip Cookie Sticks

Preparation time: 10 minutes
Cooking time: 28 minutes
Servings: 4

Ingredients:

- 1 tbsp melted butter
- 1/8 tsp vanilla extract
- 1 tbsp sugar-free maple syrup
- 1 egg yolk
- 1/8 tsp baking powder
- 3 tbsp almond flour
- 1 tbsp unsweetened chocolate chips

Directions:

1. Preheat the waffle iron.

2. Add all the ingredients to a medium bowl and mix well.

3. Open the iron and pour in a quarter of the mixture. Close the iron and cook until crispy, 7 minutes.

4. Remove the chaffle onto a plate and set aside.

5. Make 3 more chaffles with the remaining batter.

6. Cut the chaffles into sticks and serve.

497. Sausage Ball Chaffles

Preparation time: 15 minutes
Cooking time: 28 minutes
Servings: 4

Ingredients:

- 1 lb Italian sausage, crumbled
- 3 tbsp almond flour
- 2 tsp baking powder
- 1 egg, beaten
- ¼ cup finely grated Parmesan cheese
- 1 cup finely grated cheddar cheese

Directions:

1. Preheat the waffle iron.

2. Pour all the ingredients into a medium mixing bowl and mix well with your hands.

3. Open the iron, lightly grease with cooking spray and add 3 tbsp of the sausage mixture. Close the iron and cook for 4 minutes.

4. Open the iron, flip the chaffles and cook further for 3 minutes.

5. Remove the chaffle onto a plate and make 3 more using the rest of the mixture.

6. Cut each chaffle into sticks or quarters and enjoy after.

498. Garlic Bread Chaffles

Preparation time: 10 minutes
Cooking time: 14 minutes
Servings: 2

Ingredients:

- 1 egg, beaten
- ½ cup finely grated mozzarella cheese
- 1 tsp Italian seasoning
- ½ tsp garlic powder
- 1 tsp chive-flavored cream cheese

Directions:

1. Preheat the waffle iron.

2. Mix all the ingredients in a medium bowl until well combined.

3. Open the iron and add half of the mixture. Close and cook until golden brown and crispy, 7 minutes.

4. Remove the chaffle onto a plate and make a second one with the remaining batter.

5. Cut each chaffle into sticks or quarters and enjoy after.

499. Pumpkin-Cinnamon Churro Sticks

Preparation time: 10 minutes
Cooking time: 14 minutes
Servings: 2

Ingredients:

- 3 tbsp coconut flour

- ¼ cup pumpkin puree

- 1 egg, beaten

- ½ cup finely grated mozzarella cheese

- 2 tbsp sugar-free maple syrup + more for serving

- 1 tsp baking powder

- 1 tsp vanilla extract

- ½ tsp pumpkin spice seasoning

- 1/8 tsp salt

- 1 tbsp cinnamon powder

Directions:

1. Preheat the waffle iron.

2. Mix all the ingredients in a medium bowl until well combined.

3. Open the iron and add half of the mixture. Close and cook until golden brown and crispy, 7 minutes.

4. Remove the chaffle onto a plate and make 1 more with the remaining batter.

5. Cut each chaffle into sticks, drizzle the top with more maple syrup and serve after.

500. Fried Pickle Chaffle Sticks

Preparation time: 10 minutes
Cooking time: 4 minutes
Servings: 1

Ingredients:

- 1 egg

- 1/2 cup mozzarella cheese

- 1/4 cup pork panko

- 6-8 pickle slices, thinly sliced

- 1 tbsp pickle juice

Directions:

1. Mix all the Ingredients, except the pickle slices, in a small bowl.

2. Use a paper towel to blot out excess liquid from the pickle slices.

3. Add a thin layer of the mixture to a preheated waffle iron.

4. Add some pickle slices before adding another thin layer of the mixture.

5. Close the waffle maker's lid and allow the mixture to cook for 4 minutes.

6. Optional: combine hot sauce with ranch to create a great-tasting dip.

CONCLUSION

I hope this book was able to help you along your keto journey. It's easy for anyone to be overwhelmed, especially when they're new to the ketogenic diet. This book has compiled a good number of recipes for one of the easiest keto-friendly foods—the chaffle.

If you have read and skimmed through this book already, the next step is to buy a waffle maker, and start gathering the ingredients you need for any recipe you wish to try.

I wish you luck in your keto journey!

Made in the USA
Monee, IL
22 August 2020